STRUCTURED HEALING

Harold I. Magoun Jr.,

D.O., F.A.A.O., D.O. Ed. (Hon)

STRUCTURED HEALING

Harold I. Magoun Jr., D.O., F.A.A.O.

Published by Harold I. Magoun Jr.
P.O. Box 1509
Vail, Colorado 81658

Cover Design by David Magoun

Produced by Full Spectrum Arts & Services
www.fullspectrumarts.com
P.O. Box 1032
Littleton, Colorado 80116

Printed by A & L Litho, Inc.
Escondido, California

ISBN 20-9708098-0-8

Printed and bound in the United States

DEDICATION AND ACKNOWLEDGMENTS

My father, Harold Magoun Sr., D.O., F.A.A.O., received numerous awards from the Osteopathic profession in return for his dedication and contributions to the profession. He achieved international recognition, including having an Osteopathic College in Lognes, France named after him. He was the author of dozens of published articles, and two books, "Osteopathy in the Cranial Field," and "Practical Osteopathic Procedures." As Osteopathy spreads throughout the world, "Osteopathy in the Cranial Field" has been translated into French, German, Italian, and Japanese,. There is little else to add to his accolades. Therefore I have elected to dedicate this book to my mother, Helen C. Magoun, D.O. who's outstanding Osteopathic career was cut short by serious illness, but in later years her health was restored by good nutrition. Though bedfast for many years, she taught me many of the values in life, and did much to encourage my professional career.

I would like to thank my many patients over the years who have complied with my advice and recommendations, and have demonstrated that even in serious conditions, by taking charge of their lives, and by utilizing Osteopathic Manipulative Treatment, their health can be improved.

I am grateful to Michael L. Kuchera, D.O., F.A.A.O. of the Kirksville College of Osteopathic Medicine, for writing the Foreword. Dr. Kuchera is a long-time friend, and has dedicated his life to Osteopathic Education.

I want to thank my long-time friend, Galen Seal Jr., Sales Manager of A & L Litho, for his technical advice, and for getting my book printed.

My son, David (Full Spectrum Arts & Services) with his extensive artistic and computer knowledge, has been of invaluable assistance in the writing and publication of this book. The book would likely not have been accomplished without his help. He also, in a critical illness, benefited from Osteopathic Treatment.

Harold Magoun, Jr., D.O., F.A.A.O., F.C.A., D.O. Ed. (Hon)

iii

PREFACE

"I am the master of my fate, I am the captain of my soul." Nowhere is this more true than in a person's potential for controlling their own health. Appropriately, these famous words were written during a health crisis by William Earnest Henley *(1)* a nineteenth century English poet, critic, and editor. Henley had tuberculosis of the bone which had caused amputation of one foot, but the other foot was saved by some radical new surgery done by Joseph Lister, M.D., the famous English surgeon, However, Henley had been forced to spend eighteen months in an Edinburgh infirmary, during which he wrote "Invictus" from which the famous lines are taken.

We cannot always avoid serious injuries, but we can avoid many of the nagging infections, the degenerative changes, the nervous and mental diseases, and probably even cancer, by maintaining good health and thereby preventing many of the ills which afflict mankind. How do we do this? We need to structure our lives for good health by getting optimum nutrition, by engaging in appropriate exercise for our age and situation, by observing good sleep habits, by promoting good mental health, by avoiding harmful substances, and by minimizing harmful environmental factors. Persons with existing health problems have the best chance of over-coming those problems by following these same guidelines. To do this requires both will-power and "won't-power," which unfortunately many people are woefully short of. It is a question of mind over matter, but sadly, too many people have not enough mind and too much matter.

The main reasons for poor health are lack of proper knowledge of how to promote good health, not structuring our lives when we know better, receiving poor advice, and persisting in bad habits. We are creatures of habit, and unfortunately they are not always good habits.

This book is not meant to be a reference text for nutrition, exercise, or other health habits, but rather it is meant to be a source information, motivation, and positive changes a person can make both to improve and to maintain good health. The information presented has been gained from fifty years of Osteopathic practice, from reading countless books and articles, from thousands of hours of post-graduate education, from extensive teaching experience, and from just common sense. My hope is that it will prove of benefit to many people. Our most precious possession is our health, and many people don't appreciate it until they start losing it.

Harold Magoun Jr., D.O., F.A.A.O., F.C.A., D.O. Ed. (Hon)

FORWARD

A visionary physician once said, "to find health is the object of the doctor, anyone can find disease." This frontier physician, Andrew Taylor Still, M.D., D.O., founded the osteopathic profession over 100 years ago in Kirksville, Missouri. It is an idea whose time has come again. Still's distinctive philosophy of health care has inspired a number of timely books including *Spontaneous Healing* by Andrew Weil, M.D., and *Touch of Life* by Robert Fulford, D.O.

Now in this book, *Structured Healing,* Harold Magoun Jr. D.O., F.A.A.O. has created a tribute to the founder of the osteopathic profession, and his revolutionary beliefs about health. It is obvious that Dr. Magoun has diligently practiced the art of Dr. Still's patient-centered philosophy for the past 50 years. Through his experience and insight, Dr. Magoun shows us the value of seeking health, while providing a framework for us to do so.

In 1892, Dr. A. T. Still established a profession whose mission it was to change the paradigm of health care delivery. He wanted his school to provide a totally new educational model that valued the patient more than the disease - a model that taught it's students to know and respect the mind, body, and spirit of each individual so that treatment could be custom-tailored to each. Still recognized that disease in an abnormally functioning body was just as predictable as health was in a normally functioning body. Thus, for him and his students, a primary treatment goal was to maximize the function of the body within it's existing structure. Today, in *Structured Healing,* Dr. Magoun strives to teach us about Still's paradigm shift - not by lecturing in historic terms, but rather by encouraging each of us to experience the shift in practical everyday living.

vi

In reading *Structured Healing*, recognize that the word "doctor" means "teacher." Like all good teachers, "Doctor Magoun" hopes to pass on underlying principles for lifelong learners to use in shaping their decisions in the future. To this end, "Doctor Magoun" shares the value of understanding four basic osteopathic principles - the same principles that started the "health" revolution in the United States and that personally guided him in fifty years of successful patient care. Each reader recognize and seize responsibility for his or her own health, while choosing appropriate "teachers" along the way to help.

The four osteopathic tenets applied by osteopathic doctors / teachers are listed below. I urge you to seek to better understand their application as you read *Structured Healing* and to apply them as you seek optimum or high-quality health. The four tenets are:

(1) Each of us is a unit composed of mind, body and spirit each part of which is inter-dependent in maximizing true health.

(2) Within our bodies, each of us has self-healing and self-regulating mechanisms that direct our bodies toward health when given essential materials and support.

(3) Our body's structure determines how our body functions. Likewise, functional demands on our body can modify it's structure.

(4) Rational approaches to maximize health involve considering and applying the three other osteopathic tenets listed above.

It started with the vision of one man. It continues in practitioners such as Harold Magoun, D.O., who seek to be teachers of health rather than care-takers of disease; who remind us to recognize that health comes from within; who challenge us and share principles to structure health and healing in our own lives. Thank you Dr. Still and thank you Dr. Magoun.

Enjoy this book as much as I have and *seek health*.

Michael L. Kuchera, D.O., F.A.A.O.
Professor of Osteopathic Manipulative Medicine
Vice President for International Osteopathic Education and Research
Kirksville College of Osteopathic Medicine

Addendum: For his past service, insights, and accomplishments, I had the pleasure this year as Dean of his alma mater, of awarding Harold Magoun, Jr., D.O., F.A.A.O., the honorary degree, "Doctor of Osteopathic Education." He has also been awarded the A. T. Still Medallion of Honor by his specialty college, the American Academy of Osteopathy. These are the highest honors that each organization can bestow. Dr. Magoun is an outstanding physician deserving of both.

Now 73 years old, Dr. Magoun practices what he preaches. Let us all hope this will be our individual legacy.

Michael L. Kuchera, D.O., F.A.A.O.

December 2000

CONTENTS

Section I

Structuring Your Life For Health

Section I Table of Contents

1

Nutrition

There is nothing more important to good health than good nutrition, and the only one who can control that is the person him or herself. The parent is the one to control it for the child. The late Adelle Davis, one of the early nutritionists who contributed significantly to the field said, "As I see it, each of us is responsible for his own health. Others can make suggestions, but no one except ourselves can eat the foods of value to us. The health we enjoy or the amount of sickness we must endure, therefore is largely of our own making. When one sincerely wants health and is willing to work patiently toward it, the rewards are usually forthcoming". *(2)*

Almost everyone likes to eat. We also like to eat what we like, and what we like is not always the best food for us. A healthy appetite is a good sign, while on the other hand, loss of appetite is invariably a sign of illness of some kind. A healthy appetite is very much to our advantage when we choose foods that are beneficial to us, and when we eat reasonable amounts. Every individual is not only different in their personality, their fingerprints, their DNA, but also their metabolism and food requirements. There is probably more information and more mis-information available about nutrition than any other subject. There are a multitude of so-called diets, and new ones come along with great regularity. Certain diets may be of benefit to a certain segment of the population, but not for everyone, and we need to understand our individual differences.

I had a very personal experience with the dramatic changes good nutrition can make, which left an indelible impression I have carried ever since. As noted in the Introduction, both of my parents were Osteopathic Physicians. My father's family came from New England, and my mother's family came from France and homesteaded near McCook, Nebraska. My mother's family were tubercular, and both parents and one daughter succumbed to the disease. My parents practiced in Scottsbluff, Nebraska for twelve years and then moved to Denver, Colorado so my father could take over the practice of Dr. D.L. Clark, a famous pioneer Osteopath who was dying of cancer. My mother's health was failing and she was no longer able to practice. She was suffering from tubercular glomerulo-nephritis, a severe kidney disease. She was bed-fast for many years, and was not expected to live. In the late 1940's while I was in Osteopathic College, my parents heard about Adelle Davis, the famous nutritionist quoted above. They instituted Ms. Davis's nutritional program, and after several months my mother was able to get up and lead a normal life again. She finally succumbed at 79 to other causes.

Following her example, I got on the same nutritional program, and in 50 years of practice I have not lost one day out of my office from illness. There were some days that I didn't feel quite up to par, but I was able to go to work. I have missed some time from injuries, but they always healed rapidly, so I firmly believe in good nutrition.

What is good nutrition? It is giving your body the right amounts of protein, fat, carbohydrate, vitamins, minerals, enzymes, and water necessary to have a good quality of life. It will greatly enhance one's ability to resist disease, to more completely overcome injuries, to minimize degenerative changes, and delay

4

the aging process. What more can we ask? This is not a reference book of nutrition, but rather some general truths about how good nutrition and structuring one's life in other ways can enable you to take command of your life and be the master of your fate and the captain of your soul.

There are certain basic truths which need to be understood about this human body of ours. First of all, human beings have an omnivorous digestive tract, which means that it is designed to process all, foods/proteins, fats and carbohydrates all in the same meal. Some people make it even more so by putting all kinds of junk in their stomachs that doesn't belong there in the first place. Some diet faddists recommend eating only one kind of food at a time for one meal. In instances where there is a severe digestive problem, this may be necessary, but for the average person this is not necessary. Food should be thoroughly chewed to render it into small particles, and to allow the digestive enzymes and other substances to have the optimum opportunity of completing the digestive process. Carbohydrate metabolism starts in the mouth with the action of the ptyalin in the saliva, is suspended in the acid environment in the stomach, and then is completed in the small intestine with the action of pancreatic and small bowel enzymes. Protein digestion starts in the stomach by the action of stomach acids, and is completed in the small bowel by enzymes. Solid proteins need to be thoroughly chewed to allow complete digestion, and should not be overcooked. Fat digestion is accomplished in the small bowel by the action of bile salts which have been stored in the gall bladder and released in response to oil or fat in the meal, and completed by pancreatic and intestinal enzymes. It therefore follows that fat-saturated starch such as frenchfries, donuts, and deep-fried foods are not well digested, but how many tons of french-fries are consumed each year?

The essential items in nutrition are proteins, carbohydrates, fats, vitamins, minerals, trace elements, enzymes, fiber, and water. In addition many herbs have beneficial effects, but are no substitute for vitamins and minerals. The most important substance is protein. Nearly everything in the body is protein of one kind or another. Bones are a protein framework with minerals deposited on it. Connective tissue which holds everything together is collagenous protein substances. The nervous system is made up of complex proteins. Blood cells, enzymes, hormones and genes are protein. Important constituents of the cerebro-spinal fluid and the albumin and globulin of blood serum are protein. It can be seen then that a deficiency of protein can affect every aspect of body function. Proteins are made up of many different amino acids, most of which our bodies can manufacture, but there are nine that we cannot produce and must be obtained in our diet. These are known as "essential" amino acids. Proteins that contain these essential amino acids are termed "complete," and those that don't are therefor called incomplete. Complete proteins are meat, fish, poultry, shell fish, eggs, dairy products and soy beans. The latter is the only significant vegetable complete protein. Many foods contain some of the amino acids, but vegetarians must get vegetables, nuts, and members of the bean family all in the same meal in order to get all of the essential amino acids. Most vegetarians are not really unhealthy, because being that conscious of their diet, they do not eat much of the junk foods that other people consume, but many of them are protein deficient, and unless they take a supplement, are deficient in vitamin B12, the main source of which is red meat.

According to an article which appeared in the Rocky Mountain News on June 20, 1998, Many nutritionists and some pediatricians do not feel that a vegetarian diet is adequate for children. They feel it lacks the calories and protein necessary for proper growth, and is deficient in iron. Soy beans are a good source of protein for the majority of people who are not allergic to it. Studies have shown that Asians who eat soy beans are less prone to heart disease, but the key factor may be that their other sources of protein are fish, which have unsaturated fatty acids iron, Vitamin B 12, calcium and zinc, whereas in the Western World we eat more meats which have more saturated fats, and many people don't get the nutrients necessary to metabolize the cholesterol. One of the greatest gifts you can give your children is teach them how to eat properly. I feel very strongly that many diseases considered hereditary are actually poor eating habits passed from one generation to the next.

In order to get adequate protein for tissue repair, replacement of vital substances, and maintenance of body economy, we should get some protein in each meal. Nutritionists differentiate between "live" and "dead" protein, live being the fresh food sources, which contain vitamins, minerals, and enzymes essential for good health. Dead proteins are dried food extracts or amino acid supplements, which are useful for quick protein replacement, but in long-term usage are no substitute for the more healthy "live" proteins.

Although dairy products are complete proteins and are included in many diets, they have some definite disadvantages. Milk is notorious for being mucous producing and will complicate any respiratory problem. In many people it also tends to be constipating. Milk is an alkaline solution which is why it has been so widely prescribed for stomach hyperacidity, and used as an antidote for acid poisons. As I pointed out earlier, protein must be in an acid medium in order to be digested. Some people do not have enough stomach acid to acidify milk and then complete the digestive process, so they get incomplete breakdown products from the milk and get allergic or other unpleasant reactions. Yogurt has already been acidified by the bacterial action so it is more easily digested for some people.

There is considerable confusion about so-called food allergies. Some are outright allergies, while others are just lesser intolerances. Much of the mystery has taken out of this problem in recent years, for those who will listen. In 1990 at an Osteopathic meeting in Alexandria, Virginia I heard a lecture by Richard

Power, Ph.D., an anthropologist. His research led him to believe that food tolerances are linked to blood types, which can be traced back to ancient areas of geographic origin. He feels that man has not changed physiologically in thousands of years, but as we became nomadic and spread out over the globe, new substances were added to our food chain, and in many instances we have not developed the enzymes necessary to digest them. Examples of this are milk, wheat, and corn. Ancient nomadic tribes consumed goat's and camel's milk, and what was not consumed fresh was turned into yogurt which would keep for a while without refrigeration. We all therefore can tolerate goat's and camel's milk. People with type O blood, the oldest blood type, do not tolerate cow's milk. I mentioned that both my parents were practicing physicians, so I was a bottle baby. I was allergic to cow's milk, so I was raised on goat's milk. I thought little of that until I heard Dr. Powell's lecture in 1990. I am O negative. Dr. Powell was to have published a book, but apparently didn't. In 1998 a patient told me about a book relating blood types to food intolerances. I obtained the book, "Eat Right 4 Your Type," *(3)* by Dr. Peter D'Adamo, and found he had reached the same conclusions as Dr. Powell. I believe their findings make a great deal of sense, and take much of the mystery out of food intolerances. The more negative factors we can remove from our lives, the better off we are.

Protein is the only source of the building blocks (amino acids) to promote growth, repair tissue, maintain our immune system, provide the formation of hormones and enzymes, and it supplies an efficient source of energy.

Lack of protein will adversely affect every system and function of the human body, some effects more apparent than others. One of the most visible evidences of protein deficiency is dependent edema, or swelling of the feet and ankles. Many older people, particularly if they live alone, don't cook for themselves and eat poorly. The albumin and globulin, important protein constituents of the blood serum, account for about 85% of the osmotic pressure which holds fluids within the blood vessels, and if deficient will allow fluids to escape out into the tissues where it will collect in the lowest parts of the body. Very often these people don't get exercise which complicates the problem, because the pumping action of the postural muscles during activity is the motive force which returns the venous blood and lymphatic fluids back to he heart. In such cases, heart and kidney problems need to be ruled out, but even when present, most of these persons are poorly nourished. The dependent edema will usually respond quickly to amino acid supplements and more dietary protein, and vitamin B6 will act as a natural diuretic to eliminate the excess fluid. Usually 100 to 400 mg 3 or 4 times a day will accomplish this without depleting the body of electrolytes the way the drug diuretics do. These patients can also help themselves by lying down, elevating their legs, and then gently tightening and then relaxing their leg muscles to pump the fluid back to the heart.

In younger patients, usually the first sign of protein deficiency is poor tissue tone. Good healthy tissue is more firm than poorly nourished tissue.

A very important hidden symptom of protein deficiency is weakening of the intervertebral discs. Lack of protein weakens the fibers of the disc, and alters the nucleus pulposis, the gelatinous center of the disc. The latter is a colloidal substance in which an increase in the number of contained particles will increase the pressure within the system. In lack of protein, the mucoproteins in the nucleus fragment, increasing the number of particles, thereby increasing the pressure. This along with the weakening of the fibers, makes those discs much more subject to bulging or actual rupture.

Lack of protein also weakens the immune system. This is becoming more and more important as more virulent strains of bacteria and viruses are being produced. Some of this is due to the indiscriminate use of antibiotics. For instance, too many doctors prescribe antibiotics for colds and flu, which are viral infections and do not respond to antibiotics. In bacterial infections, moderate doses of an appropriate antibiotic will act as a birth control agent for the bacteria, but it is up to the immune system to eliminate the infection. Only in large doses do antibiotics become bacteriocidal, but this destroys normal bacteria which have some important functions in the body, but also greatly increases the risk of an adverse reaction to the antibiotic. We will discuss more about resistance to infections later in the book.

Protein must not be overcooked. Heat coagulates the protein molecules and makes them less digestible. There also is some evidence that well-done or burned protein can be carcinogenic. Meat should be rare or medium-rare. Eggs should be poached or soft scrambled. The pasteurization of milk is a heat process, and renders milk less digestible.

Carbohydrates include both sugars and starches. There are several kinds of sugar. Glucose is a single molecule of sugar, a monosaccharide, found in fruits, plants, and in our blood serum. It is an important source of energy. Dextrose is another form of glucose, as is fructose which is found in fruits and honey. Sucrose is a disaccharide, or two molecules of sugar found in sugar cane, sugar beets, and sorghum. It is broken down into glucose in our digestive tract. Cane and beet sugar is the purest chemical produced in such vast quantities in the world. The average consumption of sugar in this country is 100 pounds per person per year. Sugar provides energy, but no nutrients, and because it's metabolism requires nutrients, it then contributes to nutritional deficiencies.

Starches are multiple sugars which must be broken down to glucose in the digestive process. This is why starch held in the mouth for 15 to 20 minutes will start turning sweet as it is broken down to sugar by the action of ptyalin in the saliva. Natural long chain carbohydrates or starches have nutritional elements and fiber, which are both an important source of energy and form essential bulk in the intestinal tract. Some manufacturers take wheat, remove the natural nutrients, bleach it with a substance that is considered toxic by some nutritionists which then makes white flour, they add a few synthetic vitamins and call it "enriched flour." This is utter nonsense.

In response to the ingestion of sugar, the pancreas secretes insulin to convert the sugar to glycogen for energy. What isn't burned as energy is turned into storage fat. The more rapidly sugar is absorbed, the more rapidly this conversion system is activated.

In time with frequent activation, the mechanism can get "trigger happy" and over-respond, which can lead to either hypo-glycemia, or in susceptible individuals to diabetes. As blood sugar drops, we tend to crave more sugar, and many people naturally respond by consuming more sugar in the form of a soft drink, a candy bar, or some other form of sugar, which then starts a vicious cycle. Adequate protein intake tends to stabilize the blood sugar so we don't crave more sugar. So protein snacks are much healthier.

We all have a natural sweet tooth, but many people now recognize that this is harmful to our health, and some nutritionists consider sugar a slow acting poison. So in response to this a number of sweeteners or sugar substitutes have been produced, many of which appear to have long-term harmful effects. So people are torn between big bad sugar and possible harmful effects of the substitutes. Why not take charge of your life and curb your sweet tooth? It is good for your health and a good exercise in self-control. I have long maintained that on an adequate protein diet, an occasional sweet treat is not harmful. Recent research is indicating that this is true.

Many nutritionists feel that sugar is particularly bad for kids in many ways including affecting their behavior, and I agree. This concept is resisted by many doctors. Many businesses feel they are being really "good guys" by giving a child a sucker as a treat. That is totally wrong.

Starches form a large part of the average American diet. Part of the reason is that starches please the palate of many people. However I feel a major reason is that refined starches are cheapest food available, so people with limited income buy mostly starchy foods. Unfortunately this is very poor economy, because it leads to poor health and the distinct possibility of more doctor bills.

Natural long-chain carbohydrates, whole grains and vegetables, as I have already stated, have nutritional substances and fiber which are essential to our health. With the exception of vitamin C in citrus fruits, all other vitamins and minerals are found primarily in vegetables and meats. Most vegetables are nutritionally deficient today due to soil depletion, artificial fertilizers, and processing for convenience of shipping and storing rather than to preserve the nutritional value. Foods are more apt to be deficient in minerals, because they manufacture the vitamins as they grow and mature, but they must extract the minerals from the soil, which too often is deficient in minerals and trace elements.

Continued consumption of refined sugars and starches invariably leads to degenerative diseases such as arthritis and fibromyalgia, recurrent infections, deterioration of the nervous system, and an inferior quality of life. When at a super market look in the basket of a person crippled with arthritis, wearing thick glasses, fitted with false teeth, and you will likely see white bread, packaged cereals, donuts, potato chips, and other refined foods.

Many athletes practice "carbohydrate loading" before demanding athletic events. This is an acceptable practice which gives them extra energy, but should only be done occasionally.

This has only touched the surface of the importance of the right carbohydrates, the drawbacks of wrong carbohydrates, and some common sense about how to improve one's health. There are many good books on nutrition which will offer more details in this regard.

Fats and oils. In recent years, fat has been saddled with a bad reputation which is largely unjustified. Fats have been blamed for elevated cholesterol and heart disease, and to a limited extent that is true, particularly in the absence of some essential nutrients necessary to metabolize fats. However, the situation is more complicated than that in light of recent discoveries.

Fat is absolutely essential to our well-being. It is a major source of energy, much more so than carbohydrate, not only from direct ingestion of fat, but both protein and carbohydrate are converted into storage fat in the presence of certain nutrients, lecithin being one of the more important ones. Fat is stored in two major ways in the body, in the liver as triglycerides, and in various fat deposits throughout the body. These fat deposits act as padding for some organs, act as insulation, and contribute to the rounded contours of the body. In proper amounts this can be quite attractive, especially in the female, but in excess amounts can have quite the opposite effect. It has long been thought that excess fat was always detrimental to health, but this is being proven as not always true. The digestion of ingested fat is started in the small intestine by the action of bile, which contains water, lecithin, cholesterol, minerals, acids, and pigments, and then completed by the action of digestive enzymes from the small bowel and the pancreas. Bile is stored in the gallbladder where it is stored and concentrated for use in response to fat and oil in a meal. On a diet deficient in fat, the gallbladder is not stimulated to empty which can result in the formation of gall stones, usually cholesterol or pigments. It also impairs the absorption of the fat-soluble vitamins, A, D, E, and K, and what little fat has been ingested. Stones are also more likely to form in a deficiency of vitamin E.

Digested fat is reduced to fatty acids, glycerol, lecithin, vitamin B6, choline, inositol, and magnesium. This illustrates the importance of both vitamins and minerals in the digestive process. In the liver fat is broken down to fatty acids and triglycerides for energy, and to synthesize cholesterol and phospholipids.

Cholesterol, phospholipids, and triglycerides are termed lipids, meaning fatty substances, and are extremely important. Some cholesterol is contained in dietary fat leading to it's bad reputation, and is termed exogenous cholesterol. Much more cholesterol is manufactured in the body, termed endogenous, mostly in the liver, but also in many other tissues. Some is formed by the action of sunlight on vitamin D in the skin. Cholesterol forms an important constituent of cell walls, is used to make hormones of the adrenal glands, ovaries and testes. When metabolized it breaks down into cholic acid and bile salts, and then is recycled. Cholesterol exists in several forms, termed LDL or low density lipoprotein, MDL or medium density lipoprotein, and HDL or high density lipoprotein. Excessive amounts of LDL leads to deposits in the walls of arteries, where the crystals coalesce, then fibrous tissue invades the area leading to plaque formation, which can later become calcified and cause blockage of the vessel, or weaken the wall and lead to rupture with hemorrhage. HDL appears to absorb extra cholesterol crystals, thus helping to prevent heart attacks. Recent evidence would indicate that along with elevated LDL, an excessive amount of the amino acid homocysteine causes clumping of blood platelets and damages the vessel walls, and may be the real culprit in heart attacks. Homocysteine is used to manufacture protein and to facilitate metabolism. Excessive amounts can be controlled by vitamin B6, B12, and folic acid in the diet.

Phospholipids are the third group of lipids and are formed by fatty acids and phosphoric acid. Lecithin is one of the more important of this group, and can be said to act as a detergent for fats and oils. It is absolutely essential for burning fat, and necessary in any weight loss program. Phospholipids have important structural uses in cell membranes, are involved in blood clotting, and are important in the myelin sheath which insulates nerve fibers. Thus they are important in diseases of the nervous system.

It has long been known that man has a "sweet tooth", but

more recently scientists have decided that man also has a craving for fat, or a "fat tooth." Because fat has been associated with obesity, not altogether true, and associated with heart attacks, not altogether true, a fat substitute has now been produced so mankind can satisfy his "fat tooth." This should cause some concern because it does not allow for the absorption of the fat soluble vitamins and is bound to lead to health problems. Come on folks, take charge of your life!

Because of their fat content and it's commonly supposed association with elevated cholesterol and obesity, red meat and eggs have received bad publicity in recent years. This is too bad because both are good sources of protein if lecithin, unsaturated fatty acids, and choline from vitamin B complex are available for their metabolism. Organically grown beef, and farm fresh eggs where chickens can eat natural foods and be exposed to sunlight, have these nutrients in them. Farm fresh egg yolks have a rich golden color, whereas the common mass-produced eggs of chickens kept in cages, fed by conveyor belt, and not exposed to sunlight have a pale yellow color, do not contain the natural nutrients, and do not have the flavor of natural eggs. They even cook differently, which I learned several years ago when I bought a microwave and accepted the offer of a microwave cooking class with the purchase. Our instructor said that farm fresh eggs cook more rapidly than the mass-produced ones, but didn't know why. Undoubtedly it is due to the difference in nutrients contained therein.

Oils, both fish oils and vegetable oils, contain unsaturated fatty acids which are very important to our health. They get their name from an unused or unsaturated carbon bond in their chemical makeup. This carbon bond oxidizes easily at room temperature, and even more quickly at higher temperatures used in cooking, which turns the oil rancid, and destroys it's nutritional value. So manufacturers have hydrogenated these oils to prevent spoilage, but this too destroys the nutritional value. So natural oils should be kept refrigerated to maintain the nutritional value. Margarines, "creamy" peanut butter, and similar foods are hydrogenated oils and should be avoided. In natural peanut butter, the oil separates on top, and it is inconvenient to stir it back in, but it is a good source of both protein and unsaturated fatty acids. The oils essential to our health have several types of unsaturated fatty acids. The two most important are the omega 6 oils gotten from many vegetable sources such as Evening Primrose, cold-pressed olives, safflower, canola, soybeans, and the omega 3 oils from fish, especially cold water fish, and flax (linseed). Both sources should be a part of one's nutritional program. Oils are absolutely essential for lipid metabolism, for the manufacture of prostaglandins which are glandular substances with many important functions, and in recent years it has been found that the omega 3 oils have natural anti-inflammatory effects.

Many people avoid oils because of their high caloric content, but this is a mistake, and calories should be eliminated from other sources if that is one of their problems. Acne, a common and distressing problem of adolescence, in which the oil glands of the skin become clogged and then infected, will usually respond to vegetable oil, lecithin, vitamin B complex, and vitamin A. Also fat saturated starches such as french-fries should be avoided.

Fats and oils are commonly associated with obesity, as are large amounts of sugars and starches. Many people make a point of eating fruit thinking it is healthy, but over-look the fact that fruit is mostly sugar. With the exception of vitamin C in citrus fruits, most other vitamins and minerals are found in meats and vegetables. There is growing concern about the increase in obesity, which according to the Center for Disease Control and Prevention is increasing 1% per year *(4)*. There is an interesting geographic distribution with a higher incidence in the mid-west and south, and the lowest incidence in Colorado and Hawaii. The CDCP had no explanation for the geographic differences, however some logic might offer at least a partial explanation. In order to effectively reduce weight one must combine changes in diet with active exercise to burn calories. The hot humid climate of the mid-west and south are not conducive to strenuous physical activity for most people. On the other hand, the median temperatures and beautiful blue waters of the Pacific Ocean encourage more physical activity. The dry climate in Colorado and the availability of outdoor activities encourage such activity, and indeed many people migrate to Colorado just for that reason. Certainly the mile high altitude requires the expenditure of more energy which burns more calories. However, this is not a simple matter of just being fat or not. People are born with blueprints in their genes for being short, tall, large and small, and the thousands of ways we are different. Scientists are discovering many of the mysteries of our genes which explain some of these things. But then our mother's health while we are in utero will have some bearing on what happens to us later in life, and the myriad of things that happen as we grow up can affect our endocrine system which controls our size. I strongly feel that many health problems which are often considered hereditary, are actually poor dietary habits we learn from our parents.

Psychological problems are an important factor and can lead to over-eating. Recent evidence would indicate that some people are actually happier and therefor healthier when over-weight.

In 1997 Laura Fraser published a book "Losing It : America's Obsession With Weight and the Industry That Feeds It." *(5)* She put a whole new light on the subject and called attention to a more rational approach to the subject.

A number of years ago when Bariatrics, the medical practice of weight loss, became popular, a doctor friend of mine invited me to several seminars held in Denver put on by one of the companies involved in that program. Many of the lectures by endocrinologists and physiologists were very interesting, but they kept stressing the fact that Bariatrics was a legitimate practice, and a good money-maker. The latter did not appeal to me as the proper motivation for medical practice. My friend was a real ball of fire for a while. He was practicing what he preached and was taking 20 grains of thyroid a day, when usually 1 grain is an adequate dose for most hypothyroid conditions. He died of a heart attack while on vacation.

If weight is a problem, a person should concentrate more on girth or body measurements than on the weight itself. Good solid tissue from adequate protein intake and proper exercise, weighs more than flab does. We will discuss exercise in a later chapter. Usually the first place the extra flab deposits is around the waist, and we find our that "belt has shrunk." Many years ago when ski clothes were designed to be skin tight I had a lady patient who was having trouble getting into some of her clothes. I was trying to be sympathetic and said I was having trouble getting into some ski pants. She replied, "yours?"

Fiber is another important element in our nutrition and is receiving more attention. There is a story about a couple who were avid golfers. They died and went to Heaven, and were overjoyed when St. Peter ushered them into a beautiful townhouse set on a fabulous golf course with the option of playing any time they so desired, which they proceeded to do. Every shot was perfect and they knew they were indeed in Heaven. By the third day the wife noticed that her husband was getting more and irritated, but he didn't say anything. She finally asked him, "Honey, what is the matter? Here we are in this beautiful place, no cares, playing perfect golf, what in Heaven's name is wrong?" He replied, "you and your high fiber diet -- we could have been up here several years ago!" Fiber does not quite have that much impact, but is essential. Fiber is obtained only from plant sources, mostly vegetables, and some fruits, but not from meats, sea food or dairy products. It has long been known that fiber adds bulk to the stool, and with proper fluid intake will help bowel elimination. The right kind of fiber will slow down diarrhea and give the body time to process and absorb important nutrients that would be lost if the passage time is too quick. More recently it has been found that fiber absorbs harmful substances, decreases cholesterol, lowers the incidence of cancer, and reduces inflammatory disease of the bowel. There is no question but that the increase in degenerative diseases and inflammatory bowel disease in the last few generations has been due to the marked decrease in availability and consumption of natural sources of fiber. One significant factor is the decline in home gardens, a good source of natural fiber. And with more and more working mothers, more families depend on fast foods, and these highly refined foods have very little fiber in them. Again the processing of foods for convenience of shipping and storing contributes to the problem, although some manufacturers are becoming more aware of the problem and taking steps to correct it. Adequate fiber intake will help satisfy the appetite, slow down the absorption of sugar, and help in weight reduction.

Liquid intake is of vital importance, and there is no substitute for water. With coffee, tea, pop, fruit juices and other liquids, even though they are dissolved in water, there are substances the body must eliminate, and many times unwanted calories.

Water has some very unique properties, and is the most complex of all familiar substances. Under normal atmospheric conditions it can exist as a vapor, a liquid, or a solid with unusual changing properties. As it freezes into a solid, it becomes lighter than in it's liquid state, and thus floats, which in all but small bodies of water preserves the plant and animal life below the surface. Ancient man named water as the first of the four elements, water, fire, earth, and air. Our terrestrial environment is largely water, about 70%. Of that 97.2% is in the oceans, is salty and unpalatable. 2% is contained in ice caps and glaciers, .6% in ground water, .017% in lakes and rivers, and .001% in the atmosphere. So water available for consumption is less than 1% of the world's supply, and that is shrinking and becoming more contaminated each year.

In a recent report published by the Environmental Working Group in 1994 *(6)*, the water supplies of all major water sheds, especially the Mississippi, are contaminated with pesticides and insecticides. The same report found that Colorado's water supply was among the safest because most of it comes from mountain snow melt and rain, and is not contaminated from agricultural sources.

Man can only live a few minutes without air, a few days without water, but for two or three months without food. A human embryo is 80% water, a new born is about 75%, and an adult is about 65%. Every process in our bodies is carried on in an aqueous or water medium. We must have adequate water to eliminate waste products in both our bowels and kidneys. If intake is insufficient, the body re-absorbs fluid from the stool which hardens the stool and makes it both more difficult and uncomfortable to evacuate the bowel. And the urine becomes more concentrated which can lead to the formation of kidney stones which is a very painful experience. Water is also necessary to moisten the mucous membranes of the sinuses, air passages, and lungs. Dryness there increases susceptibility to both allergies and infections, and makes the interchange of oxygen and carbon dioxide more difficult. We lose a pint of water a day through those mucous membranes just from breathing, and more than that in dry climates. Thus the use of humidifiers in dry climates is very important. If the water intake falls too low, the body starts retaining fluid which can result in edema. The answer is to consume more water, and eat more protein to help hold the water in the blood vessels.

There is growing concern about whether or not our sources of water are safe be it municipal water, wells, bottled water, rain water, etc. Some are safe, some are not. The only way to find out is to have your water tested by your State lab or Health Department. Those who drink distilled water should be sure to take a mineral supplement. Municipal water supplies have chlorine added to prevent water borne infections, but in excessive amounts can be toxic. Many also have fluorine to harden teeth, but there is increasing evidence that this is not accomplished, and that other toxic effects are resulting. What about other liquids. Remember what your mother told you -- "everything in moderation." Alcoholic beverages have water in them, but in excessive amounts, the alcohol is toxic. It must be metabolized as a part of carbohydrate metabolism, which requires nutrients, and people who drink too much are always deficient in nutrients. Coffee is another common liquid which is consumed in large quantities. The caffeine content of coffee is a well known stimulant of the nervous system. People who don't eat properly very often need a "jump-start" in the morning, or a pick-up later in the day. In addition to stimulating the nervous system, caffeine also stimulates the release of adrenal hormones, elevates blood pressure, makes heart muscle more irritable, causes changes in circulation, stimulates stomach acid which can lead to ulcers, has a diuretic effect causing a loss of nutrients, contributes to elevated cholesterol, and is a common cause of insomnia, to mention some of it's drawbacks. One can eliminate the caffeine with decaf of course, but the aromatic oils which give coffee its flavor and aroma are irritating to the lining of the stomach and can cause reflex soreness in the middle of the back. Tea has as much caffeine as coffee, but the tannic acid can be soothing for some types of stomach upset. Herbal teas have many beneficial ingredients, but should be consumed only in addition to adequate water intake. Pop has many drawbacks, and yes I consume some. Many have caffeine, some have sodium which can have adverse effects, many have corn syrup for sweetening. People with type O blood, the most common type, are intolerant to corn. It is hard to find anything with sweetening that doesn't utilize corn syrup. What about fruit juice? People who drink orange juice for vitamin C are not getting what they think they are. Most of the vitamin C complex in citrus fruits is in the white pulp under them skin. In freshly squeezed orange juice, if it is not drunk within 20 minutes, 80% of the ascorbic acid has oxidized and is lost. Cranberry juice has some vitamin C, and will acidify the urine which is helpful in urinary tract infections. Recent research by Dr. John Folts at the University of Wisconsin Medical School *(6)* has indicated that purple grape juice has some anti-clotting properties due to the presence of natural substances called flavonoids. So it appears that purple grape juice may help prevent heart attacks. This is another instance where natural substances are beneficial to health. So get your 8 to 10 eight ounce glasses of water a day, and use other liquids for an occasional treat.

VITAMINS

There is probably no other area of nutrition where more misinformation is forthcoming than in vitamins as nutritional supplements. Natural foods contain vitamins, minerals and enzymes because those natural elements are absolutely essential for the metabolism of all of our foods, protein, fat and carbohydrate. I shake my head in disbelief when some product is advertized on TV with some purported nutritional benefit, and they tell you to ask your doctor. That unfortunately is too often the worst source of nutritional information. There are outstanding exceptions to this of course. Four examples that immediately come to mind are Andrew Weil, M.D., author of several books including the best-seller "Spontaneous Healing" *(7)*, Robert C. Atkins, M.D., author of "Nutrition Breakthrough" *(8)*, and a monthly newsletter, "Health Revelations" *(9)*, William Campbell Douglas, M.D. author of "Second Opinion" *(10)*, and Julian Whitaker, M.D. author of "Health and Healing" *(11)*. Tragically many doctors are ignorant of the importance of nutritional supplements. Some will mumble something about eating a "balanced diet," others will say you don't need them, and others will say you are just flushing them down the toilet. I have long maintained that if I give my body an excess of nutrients, it is better to flush some down the toilet than make my body labor under a deficiency. This approach has kept me at work every day for 50 years. If the doctors who speak against nutritional supplements would just go back and read their textbook on physiology which they had in their sophomore year in medical school, they would be ashamed that they forgot such an important aspect of their training. Even though most Medical Schools don't teach courses in nutrition, the information is all there in physiology.

As I mentioned in my opening remarks, this book is not meant to be a reference book on nutrition, but I would like to delineate some of the more important needs of the various vitamins and dispel some of the fallacies that exist.

Vitamin A. Many people are afraid to take even adequate doses of vitamin A because of the so-called liver toxicity. Vitamin A is a fat soluble vitamin and is stored in the liver, which is why liver is a good source of the vitamin. If the liver is overloaded with vitamin A, it cannot metabolize food, hence the person suffers. In mild cases it results in lethargy and weakness. In more severe cases it can cause thinning hair, aching joints, blurred vision, and flaky skin, but this does not constitute a poisoning which one would think of with the term "toxicity." The 10,000 units a day the FDA recommends is the smallest amount that will "prevent an obvious deficiency" of vitamin A. If you lived in the dark like a mushroom, and breathed filtered air you could get by that way, but that is not the way life is. I have only seen one case of so-called vitamin A toxicity. This was a young lady who was taking 250,000 units a day for acne. When the acne cleared up she kept on the same amount, but as soon as the dosage was cut back she was fine. Some skin clinics give 800,000 to 900,000 units a day for three weeks for psoriasis, which is a stubborn skin condition. By the third week the skin has usually cleared up and the dosage can be reduced. Nutritionists say you can safely give

200,000 units a day for prolonged periods without any problem. I have taken 100,000 to 150,000 units a day for 50 years. I have no allergies, rarely have colds, and have excellent night vision, the lack of which is the first sign of vitamin A deficiency. The thing I notice the most though is when skiing in the so-called flat light when it is snowing and difficult to distinguish the snow from clouds. I have better vision than other skiers.

The primary need of vitamin A is the visual process, and the cellular components of the eye. It is also important for other epithelial tissues, referring to the embryologic origin of the tissues -- the skin, hair, nails, tooth enamel, and mucous membranes which line the respiratory tract, the digestive tract, and the urinary tract. Vitamin A will help prevent and reverse cataracts, will help chronic infections of the mucous membranes such as sinusitis, colitis, cystitis, and vaginitis. It will markedly moderate allergies. It is also important for the synovial membranes which line all joints, which is why it helps arthritis. Many years ago, Alexander wrote the book, "Arthritis and common Sense" *(12)*. His mother suffered from arthritis, and after a number of doctors had failed to help her, Alexander discovered that she got significant relief from vitamin A. Being fat-soluble, he theorized incorrectly that the vitamin A was lubricating the joints, and wrote his book on that premise. His reasoning was wrong, but he helped thousands of people. However, the medical profession, instead of correcting him and learning from his example, absolutely crucified him. Joints of course are lubricated by watery synovial fluid, but vitamin A is important for the synovial membranes.

Vitamin A is also essential for protein synthesis, building and repairing cell walls, especially mucous membranes, for the immune system, and the other special senses.

Some people feel safer in taking beta carotene, which the body converts to vitamin A, but I take straight A. People who use their eyes a lot should take adequate doses of A, at least 50 to 75,000 units per day. Fluorescent lights burn more vitamin A than incandescent lights, which in turn burn more A than natural daylight. The best sources of vitamin A are liver, butter, cream, and yellow vegetables. Vitamin B Complex. This is an appropriate term for this group of water soluble vitamins, which have a number of important functions in the body, and are all inter-related. Eleven components have been isolated which are, B1 or thiamine, B2 or riboflavin, B3 or Niacin, B5 or panto-thenic acid, B6 or pyridoxine, B12 or cyanocobalamin, folic acid, biotin, inositol, choline, para-aminobenzoic acid . They are important for the utilization of energy as we metabolize our food, are important for the function of the nervous system, nourish our hair, skin, and nails, promote good appetite and digestion, and support the formation of red blood cells. One of the major differences in the typical drug store "multi-vitamin" and the natural or organic multi-vitamin obtained from Health Food stores and other natural suppliers is in the B complex. The drug store product will contain only 4 or 5 synthetic B vitamins, where the natural ones contain all 11, and we need all of them. Each of the B vitamins has some specific effects, for example B1 helps your appetite, B2 helps assimilate iron, B3 is a good vaso-dilator to improve circulation, B6 acts as a natural diuretic, B12 helps anemia, and choline is important in cholesterol metabolism. These are just a few examples, but when taken for specific therapeutic effects, basic amounts of all the B vitamins should be taken.

B vitamins are depleted by cooking, alcohol, coffee, tobacco, and stress.

One of the first signs of B complex deficiency is usually redness of the tongue and cracking at the corners of the mouth. It will also cause digestive disturbances, fatigue, and problems of the nervous system. It is a good supplement to take regularly because of it's anti-stress qualities. The best natural sources of B complex are wheat germ, brewer's yeast, and rice polishing which is the husk ground off of brown rice to get white rice. B complex should be taken in divided doses during the day because being water soluble it is not stored as well as the fat soluble vitamins. Vitamin C complex. There are several components of the C complex which are ascorbic acid, hesperidin, rutin, and the bioflavonoids. As with the B complex, the drug store Vitamin C is usually just ascorbic acid, which has some benefits, but not as much as the whole complex. Other mammals manufacture their own vitamin C, but as man evolved he did not develop that ability and must take it as a supplement.

Vitamin C is extremely important for the immune system, because without it we cannot manufacture white blood cells. This is becoming more important because of the super strains of bacteria which have been produced by the indiscriminate use of antibiotics. Studies a number of years ago that reported vitamin C to be ineffective in combating infections were erroneous because they used only a few hundred milligrams of vitamin C which are not therapeutic doses. In severe infections, a 1000 mg of vitamin C can be given every hour around the clock, because there are no toxic effects. Some people may get stomach or bladder irritation because of the acidity, so large amounts of water should also be given.

Vitamin C is important for all connective tissues -- fascias, tendons, ligaments, muscles, and the walls of the blood vessels. It will help wound healing, both surgical and traumatic, it will help strains and sprains heal, and will help prevent bruising. It helps prevent hardening of the arteries, along with other nutrients. It is a good anti-oxidant to counteract the free radicals which cause damage to our tissues. It helps delay the aging process both in the connective tissues and the brain, and will help prevent frostbite.

Vitamin C is depleted by aspirin, smoking, alcohol, air pollution, heavy metal poisoning, and many drugs. Probably the depletion of vitamin C by aspirin was a large part of Reye's syndrome, because so many doctors prescribe aspirin in fevers, not remembering that a fever is the body's natural response to an infection.

The best natural sources of vitamin C complex are citrus fruits, acerola, and wild rose hips which is the pod which develops after the bloom fades. The best part of the vitamin C in citrus fruits is in the white pulp under the skin, which usually goes down the disposal. Adelle Davis *(2)* recommended peeling the outer oily skin with a paring knife, juicing the fruit in a blender, and then drinking it within a short time. Therapeutic amounts can best be gotten in concentrated table form.

Vitamin D. This vitamin is important for bone growth and strength, for normal heart action, for function of the nervous system, and the development of the eyes. It is found in fish oils, and is produced by the action of ultra-violet on cholesterol in our skin. Deficiencies will lead to weak bones, and by affecting calcium levels will predispose to heart irregularity. Care should be taken because too much exposure to ultra-violet light can cause skin cancer.

Vitamin E. This is one of the more important vitamins. It improves the utilization of oxygen in the body thereby lessening the strain on the heart and prolonging cell membrane life, it stabilizes the hormone systems, it controls scar tissue and thus delays the aging process and is of significant help in treating burns, it is an important anti-oxidant and helps prevent the formation of free radicals, it controls fibrin which is involved in the clotting mechanism and causes blood clots, and helps protect against ozone. It promotes the maturation of the epiphyses which are the growing areas of bones, and deficiencies have been implicated in exceptionally tall people where the long bones don't stop growing.

Vitamin E is a fat soluble in most sources, which are vegetable oils, wheat germ, and some whole grains. There are some water soluble sources found in some vegetables.

Vitamin E is destroyed in cooking, by inorganic iron salts

such as ferrous sulfate which is a common iron supplement, by radiation, and by "the pill."

Vitamin K is primarily involved in the clotting mechanism, and when deficient will lead to uncontrolled bleeding. New born infants are particularly apt to be deficient if their mother was not well nourished, and can contribute to some of the complications of the newborn. The best source of vitamin K is our own intestinal bacteria, but is also found in liver and green leafy vegetables.

MINERALS AND TRACE ELEMENTS

There are many minerals and trace elements which along with the vitamins are absolutely essential for the utilization of our food, the maintenance and repair of all our various tissues, and the formation of enzymes, hormones, neurotransmitters, and the myriad of substances which make up this marvelous mechanism, the human body. I will not delineate each one of them because there are many books on nutrition which contain that information. But I must say this. I have pointed out the importance of taking nutritional supplements. In natural foods, the vitamins, minerals, and trace elements occur together. Plants manufacture their natural vitamins as they grow and mature, but must extract the minerals and trace elements from the soil. With depleted soils and artificial fertilizers, they are much more apt to be deficient in the minerals and trace elements, so their supplementation becomes even more important.

Recent evidence shows that many persons are deficient in sulfur, probably due to soil deficiencies. A good supplement for this is methyl sulfonyl methane or simply MSM, available at most health food stores. It appears to help healing in many inflammatory conditions.

I have also pointed out the inter-relationship of all the nutritional elements. This makes so-called nutritional research very difficult if not impossible. Researchers try to focus on one substance as they do in drug research, and it just doesn't work. Even when clinically successful over long periods of time, you still hear the same old story, "there is no scientific proof."

HERBS

There are literally thousands of herbs which have medicinal benefits. They have been used for time immemorial. And again we heard the same old story, "there is no scientific proof." But that is changing, and a great deal of research is being done which proves their efficacy. Perhaps the first was garlic, which now has a firm place in "alternative medicine." I will not delineate all the various herbs, that would fill a book in itself. It must be pointed out though, that even though herbs have beneficial effects, they do not replace vitamins and minerals, they are just helpful adjuncts. One important product should be mentioned though, and that is the powerful anti-oxidants, the pycnogenols, derived from grape seed and certain pine bark. These are becoming more important with each passing year because of all the noxious substances we are exposed to air pollution, chemicals, radiation, allergens, drugs, sprays, etc. We will discuss this more later when we talk about the environment.

2

Exercise

M otion is the essence of life, whether it be the whole body, an individual limb, a muscle, the blood, the lymphatic fluid, or the brain and cerebro-spinal fluid. Not too many years ago, mothers of newborn babies were kept in bed for two weeks after birth, and they got so weak they could hardly take care of their babies. Women of primitive tribes, when the time came, would squat down, deliver their baby, wrap it up, and go on about their business. So our modern women are now gotten up, and most go home the next day unless there are complications of some kind. Then it was discovered that surgical patients healed better and had fewer complications if they were gotten up, and "early ambulation" became the byword. Then it was found that even heart patients did better with motion and light exercise. In more recent years, a significant amount of research has shown that mild to moderate athletic injuries heal more rapidly if they are used and exercised. More severe injuries are kept in motion twenty-four hours a day by CPM, constant passive motion machines. Why is this? It is because for healing to take place, there must be adequate circulation. At rest, circulation is at a minimum. Essential nutrients are not carried to all body parts, waste products build up, and blood clots are more likely to form. Motion relieves nervous tension, improves elimination of waste products, and improves function generally.

One of the most basic and important aspects of motion is stretching. All four-legged animals stretch when they get up from lying. Our intelligence has blocked out that important instinct. We should stretch when we get up in the morning, but most people just get up and get going, and complain about being stiff. We should stretch before any planned exercise program or sports activity. Well trained athletes know this, as do personal trainers, many physical therapists, and exercise instructors. And we should stretch again at bedtime to help take some of the tensions of the day out before we attempt to go to sleep.

There is the story about the older gentleman who consulted his doctor one Monday morning, wanting a complete check-up, because his sexual activity was declining and his wife wasn't very happy about it. The doctor checked him carefully, took a lengthy history, and then said, "Bill, you are in good health, you are eating okay and taking your vitamins, but you are just not getting enough exercise. Starting this afternoon, I want you to start walking five miles a day, and then call me at the end of the week." So Bill did as he was told, and at the end of the week called his doctor to report. The doctor asked if he had followed instructions, to which Bill replied that he had, and the doctor then asked how his sex life was. Bill replied, "How do I know, I'm 25 miles from home!"

Ordinarily, the best exercises are natural movements such as walking, running, and swimming, provided the musculo-skeletal system is fairly normal structurally. We will discuss that in Section Two concerning the structure-function relationship of the human body. The amount and type of exercise which will be beneficial varies considerably not only in different individuals, but in the same individual from day to day depending on a many factors. These include the person's general health, any physical limitations, weather conditions, the amount of stress one is under, dietary indiscretions, environmental factors etc. Walking, running, and swimming are exercises which mobilize the body bilaterally and rhythmically, which is ideal. Persons with some impairment should walk slowly and be as relaxed as possible. They should do some deep breathing to enhance relaxation and compensate for the lack of aerobic activity. Those in better shape can "power walk" which provides a greater amount of exercise in a shorter period of time, and becomes more aerobic to inflate the lungs and encourage the exchange of oxygen and carbon dioxide. It is my feeling that when possible time wise, two or three short sessions of exercise are more beneficial than one long one. In bad weather, the treadmill offers walking exercise indoors, and many health clubs have them in conjunction with other exercise machines. Nordic Track type devices also offer rhythmic bilateral type of exercise, with more involvement of the upper body. Walking is good exercise, but involves primarily the lower body, so I have my patients who cannot engage in more active endeavors, do a respiratory stretch. With the elbows bent and the arms shoulder high, the arms are stretched back as far as is comfortable. This by means of muscle pull elevates the upper ribs, which are just used in strenuous activity. Then you take twelve to fifteen deep breaths, after which, still holding the arms up, you carefully roll the head around several times, both clockwise and counter-clockwise. This is also a good stretch for persons who sit at a computer all day.

Running, for those in good physical shape, is good exercise. This may be in the form of slow jogging, faster running, and running or jogging interspersed with short sprints. Again the amount should be varied depending on that persons status on that day. Some coaches have their athletes run up and down stairs. This is strenuous exercise, and should only be done by those in good condition.

Skipping rope is good physical activity whereby a good amount of exercise can be obtained in a short amount of time, with the added advantage of mobilizing the whole body. It should be done lightly up on the toes to prevent the pounding of the low back which occurs if done flat-footed.

In many respects swimming is the ideal exercise because it mobilizes the whole body, and the water supports the weight thus negating the force of gravity. The water should be warm enough to be comfortable, and one should swim a variety of strokes to utilize different muscle groups. For those with a stiff neck, they can use a snorkel, available at all sporting goods stores, when swimming face down. For handicapped persons, water exercise is excellent. Again, the weight is supported by the water, which makes it much easier to move impaired body parts. Movements in the water should be slow and deliberate because there is more resistance to motion in the water than there is in air. Europe is much more advanced in the prevalence and availability of therapy pools for the disabled.

Bicycle riding is another good exercise where the force of gravity is at least partially counter-acted. The seat should be high enough so the knees are fully straightened out on the down stroke of the pedals. For the average person, a regular or mountain-type bike where one sits upright is better than a ten-speed bike which requires that the rider be bent over for better aerodynamics, but is a bad position for the neck.

When one is in decent shape from these types of exercise, they will be better able to enjoy and benefit from more strenuous activities such as tennis, volleyball, racquet ball, squash, softball and baseball.

Golf, which is enjoyed by millions, is lop-sided as far as swinging the club is concerned, but most of the patients I see who get in trouble, do it by bending over to tee up or retrieve their ball. It is much easier on the back to squat down. The best part of golf is the walking, but many courses require renting a cart now. When walking is permitted, a hand cart for the golf bag is best, but if carrying the bag, it should be switched back and forth between both shoulders. One of the most lop-sided sports is bowling, but is enjoyed by millions, and is available the year around. The body will usually adapt to the one-sided nature of the game, and I see few patients who cannot engage in it. Trampolines are both a form of exercise and an athletic device. I do not consider it good exercise, because in rebounding there is a good deal of compression involved which compounds what the force of gravity does to us all day long. Then in doing the acrobatics, there is a significant amount of danger involved even in well trained athletes. About thirty years ago, trampoline parlors were quite popular, but lasted only a short time because of the injuries and the high insurance premiums required of the operators.

Many people are also doing weight-lifting, both machines and free weights. This has both advantages and disadvantages. Athletes must lift weights to build strength, but many injure themselves in the process, herniated discs being fairly common. The biggest disadvantage is that again it compounds what the force of gravity is doing to us whenever in the upright position, and this is a constant adversary. This activity also tends to build bulk, and not the good functional muscle that better forms of exercise produce. Many people when suffering from a recurrent or persistent back problem think of it as a weakness of some kind, and resort to weights to strengthen their back. In reality, the chronic problem is usually due to joint restriction and fibrous changes in the muscles and fascias from the tension of stress and injuries. They will benefit much more from stretching, mobilization and heat. Many doctors and therapists prescribe ice packs for these aches and pains. The cold numbs the area and makes it feel some better temporarily, but it restricts circulation and actually delays healing. Heat for fifteen to twenty minutes at a time is much more beneficial. In acute injuries, ice will restrict bleeding and swelling, but should not be used after the swelling has subsided. Ice can also be used in the presence of very acute inflammation, but again temporarily.

In all weight-bearing activity the feet carry the whole load, and foot problems are therefore common in societies where shoes are worn. Primitive tribes who do not wear shoes do not have the foot problems that we do. Feet need to be stretched and exercised too. I have my patients do two things. First, with shoes off, point the foot down and then rotate it slowly both clockwise and counter-clockwise. Then because in the weight-bearing position, all of the strain on the toes bends them back up towards the body, I have them stand on the edge of a step or a large book with the toes off the edge, and bend the toes down repeatedly with short intervals of relaxation in between.

Every few years some new type of exercise device is promoted, some beneficial, some not. About thirty years ago there was a device called the "Slim-Jim" which was sort of an articulated chaise lounge. It afforded some stretching and mobilization, but I had a number of patients who strained their backs getting on and off the device. Several years later a device called the "Exer-Genie" came along. This was a spring-loaded capsule with several cords coming out which you pulled on in several positions. I had a number of patients who probably over-did it, but they too sprained their backs. This is not uncommon, because so often when we make up our mind to "get with it," we over-do.

Rowing machines have been around a long time, and some people benefit from them. The position required for that activity is not good for persons with low back problems however. When patients ask me about it I usually tell them that is why they used to chain them to the oars in slave galleys centuries ago.

In recent years devices and exercises which simulate stair-climbing have become popular. Climbing stairs requires lifting the body weight the height of the step on one leg, which is more strain than just supporting the weight on level ground. Persons with low back problems do not benefit from this activity, while able-bodied people usually do.

For persons with chronic low back problems, the inversion hanging devices are excellent for stretching. Initially there was some concern about persons with high blood pressure, but research has shown that there are no adverse effects. The only contra-indication is for persons who suffer from glaucoma where there is increased pressure inside the eyeball.

Speaking of the eyeball, even eyes can be exercised and thereby improve vision. Right after the turn of the century, a distinguished New York ophthalmologist, William N. Bates, M.D. developed a series of eye exercises which dramatically improved vision. He felt that eye glasses were much like the rest of medicine and only treated symptoms and didn't really get at the cause of the problem. He adamantly opposed fitting school children with glasses, became at odds with the Medical Profession and was expelled by the American Medical Association. My mother used the Bates exercises and went from not being able to read the phone book with her glasses to reading microscopic print without her glasses. Dr. Bates work has been enlarged on by Marilyn B. Rosanes-Berrett, Ph. D. in her book "Do You Really Need Glasses?" *(13)*

When a person has suffered an injury of some kind, and is attempting to resume some special activity, after healing has taken place the best rehabilitation is doing that specific activity. One should start gradually and then increase the activity to tolerance.

Handicapped persons should be encouraged to exercise. It can be life-saving. There are many sports that are now being engaged in from wheel-chairs, such as softball, basketball, volleyball, water sports and even skiing on special mono-skis. I have patient who is a dramatic example of that phenomenon. Lisa was a champion figure skater as a young woman in Canada, and toured Europe in an ice show. She became disabled in 1985 because of a vascular mass on her spinal cord. She later became paralyzed from her upper body down, and in severe chronic pain because of unsuccessful back surgery. She was told to give up and go to bed at a nationally known rehabilitation hospital, but refused to follow their advice. Had she done so she would not have survived. She determined to help herself and started exercising in her wheel chair. She developed some aerobic exercises which she called "chairobics," and has become internationally famous for her work with other handicapped persons. She has received numerous awards, including a decoration from Nelson Mandella for her work with the handicapped in South Africa, where she lived with her husband, Dr. Mel Siff, a physiatrist from 1994 to 1998. Her rehabilitation has been aided by improved nutrition, physical therapy, and Osteopathic treatment, but mostly her own motivation and perseverance. She is a shining example of what can be accomplished.

3

Sleep

S hakespeare said it best. "Sleep that knits up the ravell'd sleeve of care." (14) Sleep should be a time of rest when healing takes place, body resources are replenished, tension is dissipated, and the subconscious is free to play out it's fantasies. Sleep is defined as unconsciousness from which the person can be aroused by sensory or other stimuli. (15) There are two types of sleep, a slow wave sleep during which the brain waves on EEG are very slow, and a second called REM or rapid eye movement. The first is the most restful and occurs when we first go to sleep. Normally we shift back and forth during periods of sleep.

The average person requires about eight hours of sleep, but it appears to be more difficult to achieve this. Early in the 1900's people were getting about nine hours of sleep. Now the average is about seven, which is due to a number of factors. There are more working mothers, we crowd more recreational activities into our schedules, and there are more distractions such as TV, the internet, traffic noise, jet noise, noisy neighbors, social obligations, and just keeping up with the Joneses. These all take their toll. There are many things which interfere with sleep.

Stress: this keeps the body "up tight," muscles are tense, and the nervous system is "racing it's motor." This makes sleep almost impossible until fatigue sets in. Depression is a negative situation which again makes the nerves and muscles tense. The nervous system and the muscles are very closely associated and we refer to them as the neuro-muscular system. Lack of sleep can cause depression, so this can very easily become a vicious cycle which is difficult to break. Certain restrictions of motion in the musculo-skeletal system can also cause depression which we will discuss in Section II.

Irregular schedule: sometimes this cannot be helped in certain work situations and in travel across several time zones, but this upsets the body's inherent time clock.

Caffeine: Some people can tolerate caffeine in the evening and still sleep, but most can't. Sources of caffeine are regular coffee, regular tea, cola drinks, chocolate, and many pain medications which include caffeine to counter-act the depressing effects of pain.

Alcohol: This induces sleep for a period of one to four hours, but then has a rebound effect which causes the person to awake and makes it difficult to return to sleep.

Heavy eating late in the evening: a large meal puts increased demand on circulation and metabolism which then interferes with normal sleep mechanics. Then what food is not used for energy is turned into storage fat. The next morning the person is usually not hungry, so no breakfast is eaten which requires the body to break down storage fat for energy producing more waste products.

Tobacco: nicotine is a nerve poison and stimulant, only one of many dangers.

Strenuous exercise: Too much physical activity can "race the motor" and make sleep more difficult. Some people sleep better after sexual activity, others do not, so it is a matter of trial and error, and there are some who would rather go without the sleep. To each his own!

Vitamin B Complex: in a small percentage of people, taking

B Complex close to sleep hours will pep up the nervous system enough to interfere with sleep, but this is not common. There are two commonly recognized physical problems which interfere with sleep. These are sleep apnea where a person stops breathing for short periods, and PLM, periodic leg movement or "jumpy leg" syndrome. In both situations there are restrictions in the musculo-skeletal system which cause these symptoms. This will be discussed in Section II.

The effects of lack of sleep are numerous and are more serious than commonly realized. Increasing attention is being paid to good nutrition for optimum health, and the importance of exercise to achieving good health, but the necessity of adequate sleep is neglected. One of the more serious aspects of sleep deprivation is the impairment of the immune system. The immune system, which consists of the white blood cells and antibodies, protects the body against foreign elements such as bacteria, viruses, allergens, toxins, and if not too impaired even cancer cells. One of the problems with chemotherapy is that it damages the immune system.

This fatigue induced impairment of the immune system may be one factor in the alarming increase in virulence of both bacteria and viruses. There is growing concern about this and the possibility of more serious plagues in coming years. This problem is very vividly described by Laurie Garrett in her book, "The Coming Plague" (16) in which she describes some of the plagues we have already experienced in recent years, and the very real danger which faces us.

Lack of sleep causes depression, loss of memory, lack of concentration, and diminished motor skills, which control voluntary muscle activities. Statistics show that a sleepy driver is seven times as likely to have an accident, and sleepiness is responsible for at least 100,000 traffic accidents per year, and at least half of fatal accidents. No doubt sleepiness is also responsible for many accidents around the home.

Lack of sleep impairs the production of many important hormones in the body, promotes the deposit of more storage fat, and accelerates the aging process, probably through the release of cortisol, an adrenal hormone which is also activated by stress. People short on sleep usually drop right off when their head hits the pillow.

There are many things we can do to improve our time and quality of sleep. First of all, try to establish regular sleep habits if your work situation allows. Try to get to bed at a fairly regular hour most of the time, and an occasional "night out" won't be that disruptive. It is important to establish good sleep habits in your children which they should carry with them to adult life, just as good eating habits will benefit their health. I firmly believe that children should be in bed by eight o'clock except on special occasions. I have five grandchildren who are allowed to stay up to all hours of the night. They are very bright, but frequently sick which I attribute to impaired immunity.

The second important factor is comfort. A good support under the body is essential. A few people prefer a water bed, although the popularity seems to be declining. Fewer yet like the inflatable air beds. I prefer a traditional mattress, and I think nowadays mattress manufacturers are aware of the importance of good support, and they design and manufacture good products. Pillows are important to support the neck and head. There are dozens of pillows on the market of all different sizes, shapes, contours, and consistencies. I prefer an old fashioned feather or Dacron pillow that you can fluff up or flatten out, depending on what position you are sleeping in. If you have difficulty sleeping, it is a good idea to take your own pillow when travelling because so many hostelries have large foam rubber pillows which are not comfortable for most people. The position you sleep in also needs to be discussed. Persons with some physical problems are limited to the positions they can sleep in. This will be discussed in Section II dealing with the structure-function relationship of the human body. You hear stories that you shouldn't sleep face down because of your stomach, perhaps true on Thanksgiving after over-eating, and you shouldn't sleep on your left side because of your heart, etc. With rare exceptions I feel these are old-wives tales. You are going to turn many times during the night normally, so when you go to bed, get in the most comfortable position you can find, and leave the rest to Mother Nature.

If you get uncomfortable during the night you are either going to turn or you will wake up. Very often when people wake up stiff in the morning they think they have slept crooked or done something in their sleep, but I don't think that is the mechanism. When you go to bed with some stiffness somewhere in your back or neck, it is going to stiffen up during the night when movement is at a minimum. When you get up in the morning and move around, it then loosens up. So, as we said in the last chapter, do some stretching at bedtime to release the tensions of the day which will help you sleep better.

The best chance you have of getting a good nights sleep is to relax at bedtime, both physically and mentally. Do some stretch-ing, particularly of the neck and shoulders, and the low back if you have backaches. Do some deep breathing, which is one of the most relaxing things you can do. It is part of all meditation and stress control programs. For most people a warm bath or shower is relaxing, as is a short session in a hot tub. Hot water is one of our greatest luxuries. It is no wonder the mountain men and native Americans gathered at natural hot springs in the spring time.

A nap in the afternoon has been found to extend the life expectancy, but later in the day will make it more difficult to get to sleep.

Of great importance is relaxing mentally. Don't watch a horror or violent movie at bedtime. Even the flickering of the TV screen can stimulate the nervous system. Some psychologists feel it is not good to watch the evening news, because so much of it is devoted to bad news which has a negative effect on our mind. Why isn't there more good news? Paul Harvey, the world's most widely heard commentator, stated in an address in 1998 which was printed by Imprimis, the monthly publication of Hilsdale College, Hilsdale, Michigan, "People often say to me, 'Paul, why don't journalists and broadcasters emphasize more good news instead of tragedy, destruction, discord, and dissent?' My own network once tried broadcasting a program devoted solely to good news. The program survived 13 weeks. In Sacramento, California, a tabloid called the Good News Paper printed nothing else. It lasted 36 months before it went bankrupt. A similar Indiana tabloid fared even worse; the publishers had to give it away. Evidently the good news people say they want is news they won't buy." *(17)*

Don't go to bed mad. Practice forgiveness, it is good for you in many ways. Don't go to bed worried, leave your worries in the other room. They may not be quite so formidable when you wake up in the morning. A bedtime prayer is the answer to many problems.

Light or humorous reading at bedtime may be beneficial and relaxing for many. Play light relaxing music, or relaxation tapes with the spoken word or a sound track of the ocean or a gentle brook. Classical music is well known for relaxing even brain injured children. The heavy bass beat of rock music is not relaxing and it is not surprising that so many of it's devotees are so hyper.

There are many sleep aids. Calcium, 1000 to 1500 mg. taken at bedtime will relax the muscles. Years ago before we had the chemical muscle relaxants we gave intravenous calcium for muscle spasm and it gave dramatic relief. For people who tolerate milk, according to their blood type, a glass of warm milk at bedtime will help. There are many herbal products which aid relaxation and sleep, and adverse reactions are rare. Melatonin as a sleep aid has been somewhat controversial, but a recent study published in Clinical Pearl News *(18)* indicated a significant difference over the placebo control group.

Tryptophan, a naturally occurring amino acid has a significant relaxing effect on the central nervous system. It was used by millions of people, and many well known doctors, including Norman Shealy, who has the most famous pain clinic in the world. A number of years ago, a number of people got sick from taking tryptophan, and the FDA took it off the market. The problem was traced to a contaminated batch from Japan, but the FDA has never authorized the subsequent release of tryptophan. I will always believe that this is due to pressure from the pharmaceutical companies, because the public pays, according to a report in USA Weekend *(19)*, over 100 million a year on over-the-counter sleep remedies, and almost 2 $1/2$ billion on prescription sleep remedies. Would the almighty dollar have anything to do with this? There are several foods which contain tryptophan, the best being turkey breast, bananas, and natural peanut butter. A snack of one of those can be of help.

There is an auto-hypnosis or self administered hypnotic technic which is very effective in aiding sleep, but should not be done without training from a well-trained hypno-therapist. It consists of lying on your back, getting as comfortable as possible, and then taking each body part one step at a time : left foot, right foot, left calf, right calf and so on, concentrating on releasing tension and getting each part to completely relax. Many years ago when I was still doing an acute practice I used the procedure, but twice I got a phone call in the middle of the night and was so relaxed when I got up to answer the phone that I passed out, so I quit using it. There is a story about a man who was having trouble sleeping, went to his doctor, explained his problem, and the doctor instructed him in this auto-hypnosis procedure. The fellow went to bed early to try it and see how it worked. He had just reached the abdominal level, when his wife, misunderstanding his reasons for going to bed early, came slinking into the bedroom in a sexy nightgown. The fellow took one look at his wife, clapped his hands, and said, "okay, everybody up!"

Many people rely on sedatives, as you can see from the above figures, but this is not good because sedatives can become habit forming, they tend to wear out their usefulness, and they tend to leave the person groggy. Combined with alcohol or other drugs, sedatives can be fatal.

With so many natural, harmless remedies for sleep, it is a mistake to resort to drugs, so take charge of your life!

4

Mental Health

Mental health is quite complicated. It is a product of the inter-action of the mind, which encompasses the nervous activity of the brain such as cognition and reasoning, the psychological manifestations governing behavior, and the lesser known influences of parapsychology or extra-sensory functions of the brain. Frank Willard Ph. D., a professor at the New England School of Osteopathic Medicine, has stated that "The mind is an emergent property of a dynamic interaction between the brain and, body." *(20)* The brain is the receptor of a tremendous amount of sensory stimuli from the whole body, all of which affect brain function.

Loss of physical health is usually more obvious than loss of mental health, and persons are more apt to deny problems of the mind. When we think of functions of the mind, two names quickly present themselves, Sigmund Freud and Norman Vincent Peale. Both are world famous, are quite unique, and are exact opposites.

Freud was born in Moravia, now Czechoslovakia, in 1856. He led a troubled life, which included discrimination as a Jew. He attended the University of Vienna, and the General Hospital of Vienna which then qualified him to practice Medicine. He was interested in mental diseases, and became famous for his psychoanalysis and dream interpretation. He rejected any belief in God or an after life, stating that religion was "an infantile helplessness." He died of cancer in 1939. Many of his teachings are still controversial. He emphasized the role of sexual desires and experiences in the functions of the mind.

Norman Vincent Peale was born May 31, 1898 in Downesville, Ohio. His father was a doctor and preacher, which was fairly common in those days. The father suffered a severe health problem which was apparently cured by prayer, after which he devoted himself to the ministry, but undoubtedly recognized the importance of mental health influencing physical health, and called himself doctor of mind and spirit. This philosophy was absorbed by young Norman. He describes himself as a bashful boy with feelings of inferiority. In college he was unable to express himself verbally, but did quite well on written tests. One day one of his professors chewed him out because he had brains, but had no faith in himself. Peale was devastated, but on the way out of the building was struck by an incredible thought which changed his life. "I don't have to be this way any longer." *(21)* He asked God to take over his life, and indeed God did. Peale recognized the power we have over our own minds and well-being, and his message through his ministries, his writings, and his Foundations have reached and touched millions world-wide. He is the author of two dozen books, the most famous being "The Power of Positive Thinking" which has been a best-seller, and translated into thirty-three languages. Most of his ministry has been at Marble Collegiate Church in New York City, founded in 1623 by the Dutch West Indies Company. He emphasized the importance of a strong faith in the Almighty, the power we have to direct our own lives, and the rewards of good mental health.

Because of the body-mind relationship, the chances of having a healthy body are better if we have a healthy mind, and vice-versa, but there are exceptions. In my fifty years of practice I have seen many patients who ignored the rules of good health, and stayed in apparent good health for many years, but I think eventually it does catch up with you. On the other hand I have seen a number of para and quadriplegics with battered bodies, who were some of the most pleasant patients I have had. I have attributed this to the fact that they have problems they know they must accept, while those with lesser problems stew and fret, impatient to get better.

Mental health has a broad spectrum. Optimists have a positive attitude and generally have better health than pessimists. They feel that things work in their favor, and tend to believe that the problems we face have lessons to learn if we just look for them. Those who exercise Peale's Power of Positive Thinking have a greater chance of being healthy both mentally and physically, and being happier along with it. Then those who carry it a step further and follow Peale's example of a firm faith in their creator, have an even better chance. It is interesting to note how many scientists during the technological advances of the Second World War and the atomic age, turned to religion. Perhaps as they unraveled the secrets of the Universe it became more apparent to them that there is a supreme being or intelligence of some kind.

Having a positive attitude and a firm faith does not guarantee being healthy however. Man is the most highly developed species on this planet, and because of this has fewer regenerative powers than lower forms of life. A lizard can grow a new tail, we cannot grow new parts. When our highly specialized tissues are damaged, they are usually replaced by less functional tissue, usually scar tissue. Very often the seeds of destruction which lead to degenerative changes are sown early in life, and then the changes we can make when we get the wisdom are therefore limited. Our existence itself is quite complicated. Some are born with a strong constitution and can withstand many assaults, others have weak constitution and react to every little insult. We are subject to many different kinds of trauma, varying degrees of stress, and what we do to help or hinder our health varies greatly. What we do in the face of all these variables can make difference though, it is just in knowing what to do. This book should give you some of those answers.

Impaired mental health can manifest itself in many ways: behavioral problems, child abuse, attention deficit, substance abuse, domestic violence, depression, criminal acts, suicide, the long-recognized mental illnesses and psychoses, and many other types of aberrant behavior. A 1995 report to the United Nations by an international team of authorities (22) stated that there was an alarming increase in mental illness worldwide, but especially in underprivileged countries. The report attributed the problem primarily to the stress of wars, political upheaval, displacement of populations, and lack of treatment. With those conditions existing, undoubtedly malnutrition plays a significant role. In the United States, depression is the most common psychological problem. (23) It can manifest itself in many ways, and come on so gradually that many times it is not truly recognized. Depressed persons may have insomnia, loss of appetite, fatigue, anxiety, indecision, crying spells, drug or alcohol abuse, loss of self esteem, feelings of guilt, social withdrawal, suicidal tendencies, and so forth. It can affect both male and female, and all ages, but is most common in the older generations. According to an article in Parade Magazine in 1995 (24), 24,000 persons over the age of 65 attempted suicide because of depression, and 6,000 succeeded. That age group is 13% of the population, but accounted for 20% of the suicides. As I mentioned in Chapter I, many older people, especially if they live alone, do not cook and eat properly, and if the body and mind are not nourished, they cannot function normally. So function gradually declines and they gradually slip into depression, which all too often then is attributed to "old age." It could be reversed. Many of these persons also have musculo-skeletal problems which affect blood and nerve supply to various areas of the body causing a decline in function. Early in the 1900's an Osteopathic Physician, Dr. Arthur Hildreth, found a relationship with restriction of the first cervical vertebra, the Atlas, where the skull sits on the spine, and the fourth thoracic vertebra, between the shoulder blades, and depression. This became known as "The Hildreth Lesion". This has been substantiated by many Osteopathic physicians, myself included. We will discuss this further in Section II on the structure-function relationship of the body.

Dr. Hildreth became interested in nervous and mental disease, and at the time of the First World War opened the Still-Hildreth Mental Sanatorium in Macon, Missouri. They combined traditional medical treatment, nutrition, and Osteopathic treatment, and had an outstanding record in treating nervous and mental diseases. In 1958, Drs. John and Rachel Woods, both accomplished Osteopathic Physicians, spent a year at Still-Hildreth studying any possible relationship between mechanical disturbances of the cranial mechanism and mental disease. Their findings were published in the Journal of the American Osteopathic Association in 1961. *(25)* There is a palpable movement in the skull which accompanies the fluctuation of the cerebro-spinal fluid, observable during brain surgery. The Woods found a marked slowing of this fluctuation in severe mental disease. This will be discussed at length in Section II.

The best foundation for good mental health is good general health. The best chance for that lies in taking charge of your life, and applying the principles of good health as outlined in this book. It is helpful to have a happy healthy family life, to have sense of responsibility, and have good self esteem. In an article entitled "Treating the Body, Healing the Mind," which appeared in the Medical magazine Hippocrates *(26)*, James S. Gordon, the well known psychiatrist is quoted as saying, "a chronically depressed person's best chance at a lifelong cure is to marshal every health-enhancing tool on God's green earth - nutritious food, exercise, meditation, acupuncture, human connection - to right her body and brain chemistry rather than relying on drugs." I would add that careful Osteopathic treatment, which will be discussed in Section II, will do much to correct structural problems which greatly impair normal function of both body and mind.

Until recent years, the importance of faith and prayer in both mental and physical health has been largely ignored, scorned and even ridiculed. Bernie Siegal, M.D. in his book "Love, Medicine and Miracles" *(27)* speaks of placing a report on his hospital staff bulletin board of a study showing the beneficial effect of prayer in reducing post-myocardial infarction complications. Infarctions are blood clots in the arteries of the heart. Within 24 hours someone had written "bull shit" across it. That attitude is changing, and as with many other things, the long-standing traditional medical criticism of "there is no scientific proof" is changing. Even prayer is getting scientific studies made. In a study in "Ways and Means" published by the Mississippi Methodist Rehabilitation Center, 700 cardiac patients in the Brockton Massachusetts VA Hospital, those that had a daily visit by the hospital chaplain left the hospital on an average of three days earlier than those who didn't, at a saving of about $4000 per patient. They concluded that spiritual support was an important part of cardiac rehabilitation. Probably heart problems and cancer create more fear in patients than most other maladies. Prayer has been shown to lower heart rate, blood pressure, respiratory rate, and brain cell activity. Another study, "Can Prayer Heal?" (28), also published in Hippocrates, found that prayer heals in many different ailments, but that prayer by the patient themselves is more effective than prayer by another person. Positive affirmations based on faith, which are closely related to prayer, are also helpful.

In a 1996 article in Time Magazine, "Faith and Healing" *(29)* cited a 1995 study at Dartmouth which concluded that one of the strongest predictors of survival after heart surgery was the strength and comfort the patient got from religion.

An article in The Rocky Mountain News, *(30)* quoted a study which showed that regular church goers live seven years longer than non-attenders.

Over the years there have been a number of well known "faith healers." I will mention only one, Kathryn Kuhlman from California. Many years ago, Dr. Viola Frymann, an internationally known Osteopathic specialist, who has the Osteopathic Center for Children in San Diego, did a medical study on some of Ms. Kuhlman's "cures." Dr. Frymann *(31)* found that those patients who had a religious experience had only a temporary relief of their problem, while those who had a religious reformation had a permanent cure.

An indication of the increasing desire for building faith is the growth internationally of "The Promise Keepers" the organization started by Bill McCartney, the football coach who took the University of Colorado to national prominence.

Faith and prayer are no longer something to be ashamed of, to be ridiculed about, or to be done in seclusion. It is proving itself in all phases of medicine. Isn't that what Norman Vincent Peale and thousands of others less known have been saying for years? But in this endeavor, let God take charge. This is difficult for many of us to do.

Good mental health can bring real happiness, and like healing, can only come from within.

5

Avoiding Harmful Substances

"**M**an is the most intelligent species of life on earth, but is the only species that deliberately inhales and consumes substances he knows are harmful." *(32)* This statement was made by I. M. Korr, Ph.D., former professor of mine at the Kirksville College of Osteopathic Medicine and now a life-long friend. Intelligent human beings, in a senseless craving for "highs," gratification, escape, being "cool," and many less obvious reasons, continue to self-destruct in spite of repeated warnings and irrefutable evidence of the harmful and often fatal results. After the second World War, an international safety group studied the reactions of people in the face of impending disasters such as bombing raids, severe storms, floods, and found that about 85% of people will ignore warnings of impending disaster! How more likely they are to ignore warnings then of insidious harm, from poor diet, smoking, excessive drinking, and so forth. A study by the Robert Wood Johnson Foundation *(33)* concluded that substance abuse, cigarettes, cigars, alcohol, and drugs, kill over 500,000 Americans per year, at a total cost of 238 billion dollars, 99 billion for alcohol, 72 billion for smoking, and 67 billion for drug abuse. These problems destroy families, increase the cost of health care, overwhelm the education, criminal justice and social system, and have led to an unprecedented wave of violence. One of the worst habits a person can have, and one of the hardest to break is smoking. Many years ago in one of his very funny monologues, Bob Newhart did one on Sir Walter Raleigh reporting to Queen Elizabeth I on his return from the New World. It went something like this. "And we also brought back some large brown leaves called tobacco. What do you do with them? You roll them up, put them in your mouth, and set them on fire!" It is so ridiculous it is funny, but how tragic it is in realization. Statistics vary, but somewhere between 350 and 450 thousand people a year die from smoking in the United States, and over three million world wide. Cigarette smoking adds at least 50 billion to the cost of health care and lost wages in the United States each year.

One of my patients, Richard L. Crowther, FAIA, a nationally known architect and environmentalist, published a book, "The Paradox of Smoking" *(34)* in 1983. This was before non-smokers did not seem to have any rights at all. Since then non-smoking areas have been designated in most public buildings, in stadiums, and smoking has been banned on most airline flights. This was a long time in coming, and now the tobacco industry is being brought to task. Mr. Crowther's book is not on how to stop smoking, but on the dangers and irrationality of smoking. Some quotes from his book are as follows. "Smoking has no positive aspects." "It is a serious drug habit. Tobacco smoking is more addictive and broadly harmful than illegalized heroin. It is toxic, addictive, odiferous, intrusive, and incendiary." "Smoking is the #1 indoor polluter, the #1 cause of cancer, respiratory and heart disease, and the #1 cause of burns and fires." "Tobacco has over 3,600 chemicals, most of them poisonous." "Persons who smoke 20 - 39 cigarettes a day have a 96% higher death rate, and those that smoke 40 or more a day have a 126% higher death rate than non-smokers."

It is a great advance to have smoking banned in so many

places, because it is so unpleasant to non-smokers, but more important is the fact that the smoke that rises from lit cigarettes, cigars, and pipes, so-called "curl smoke" or "passive smoke" is even more deadly than inhaled smoke. "Curl smoke is not filtered in any way, while smoke drawn through other tobacco and of course filters is partially filtered. The EPA ranks curl smoke with asbestos and arsenic as being the most carcinogenic agents. A study published by The Washington Post and reprinted by The Denver Post *(35)* found in a study of 32,000 nurses, that women exposed to curl smoke had almost double the risk of heart attacks. Children also suffer significantly. Another study published in The Denver Post *(36)* on July 15, 1997 stated that 6,200 children die each year from their parents smoking, which results in lung infections and burns. Such children have a much higher incidence of otitis media (ear infections), and are much more liable to have cancer of the lung later in life. Mothers who smoke have babies of lower birth rate, are more susceptible to Sudden Infant Death Syndrome, and more apt to have complications. Boys of smoking mothers suffer from conduct disorders, and are more apt to become violent juvenile delinquents.

In addition to the tremendous impact on health care costs, the time lost from work, the damage from fires, the increased insurance rates from smoking, Bottom Line *(37)* published a survey which says that 2 packs a day is as expensive as maintaining a car, about $2,500 a year. Can you really afford to smoke?

Smoking and chewing have other unseen dangers. The poisonous chemicals in smoke impair the ability of red blood cells to carry oxygen to all the tissues of the body, thereby hastening the breakdown of those cells. They destroy very important nutrients, especially vitamin C, with resulting impaired immunity with slower healing, more infections, and easier bruising. It is estimated that one cigarette destroys 25 mg. of Vitamin C. It also causes more rapid mental decline in the elderly. Smoking affects both the sense of smell and taste, making food less tasteful, resulting in greater use of seasonings and condiments which are not beneficial. It is impossible to predict the staggering cost of all these harmful effects.

In an article I wrote several years ago about the cost of health care *(38)*, I suggested that instead of subsidizing the tobacco industry, the government should implement substituting other crops, but I later learned that a tobacco farmer can support his family on a small plot of ground, which he couldn't do with other crops. The almighty dollar again.

The tobacco industry has finally cracked though, and evidence is being presented that they are aware of the addictive nature of nicotine, but have hidden the reports. The revelation has led to billions of dollars in lawsuits, and most states have filed suits to help recover some of the smoking-related health care costs. At the time of this writing those suits are up to 400 billion dollars! But still the tobacco industry continues to push it's death-dealing products, targeting the younger generation, and poorly developed countries. It is tragic that the government attempts to limit the number of vitamins we take which promote health, but subsidizes the tobacco industry which causes so much death and disease, and only requires a Surgeon General's warning on tobacco. Something is wrong there.

Smoking is one of the hardest habits to break. Richard Crowther says in "Paradox of Smoking," *(34)* "it is seldom that smokers stop smoking because of logic." Certainly if logic were involved they never would have started smoking in the first place.

A survey published in "The D.O.," a magazine published by the American Osteopathic Association *(39)* stated that persons who are able to quit try at least six times before they are successful, but most people don't want to quit. I had one patient who said it was easy to quit, she had done it 15 or 16 times.

President Eisenhower, who was a patient of my father's, was a chain smoker in the army. When he was elected President of Columbia University, he felt he should stop smoking as a good example for the students. He went through the tortures of the damned, but finally succeeded. Years later someone asked him if he thought he would ever smoke again. Ike replied, "I don't know about that, but I know I'll never quit again."

In 1997, Channel 9, KUSA in Denver aired a stop smoking campaign, aimed mostly at teenagers. They offered 12 teenagers $100 if they would stop smoking. Not one of the twelve succeeded in doing so.

We doctors are falling down on the job of discouraging smoking. Smokers say they would be more motivated to stop if their doctor told them to, but only 1/3 report that their doctor has talked about it. We doctors need to take control of that aspect of our practices, and help our patients take control of their health. This is especially true of teenagers. Eighty per cent of smokers start before they are 18. Schools should not provide smoking areas because in so doing they are contributing to the delinquency of minors and are accessories "before the fact" of countless deaths. Smokeless tobacco is also very harmful, and is becoming more popular with the younger generation. In this instance, the prosecution must never rest.

Drinking. Man has consumed fermented beverages as long as recorded history, and more than likely has over-indulged during that time. In the United States we consume over 50 billion bottles and cans of beer, and 800 million gallons of wine and alcohol a year. In the older population in recent years there has been a shift to less consumption of hard liquor in favor of more wine, In the younger population, just as smoking is on the increase, so is alcohol consumption, and it has become a major problem. According to the Carnegie Foundation *(40)*, a survey of college Presidents across the country named "binge drinking" as the number one problem on todays' college campuses. I suspect that Rush Limbaugh would say that the teaching of liberalism and depreciation of moral values is a very close second. I wonder if close examination wouldn't reveal that deviation from long established values and concepts in our educational system isn't responsible for much of the irresponsibility in our youth of today. "Binge drinking" is defined as 5 drinks in a row for men, 4 for women, one or more times in a two week period. It has been found that women do not metabolize alcohol as rapidly as men so they feel the effects more rapidly, and the effects last longer. Many college students are under the legal age for drinking, but fake ID's are easily obtainable. A Harvard School of Public Health survey cited in the same Britannica article *(40)* found that in 17,000 students from 140 colleges in 40 states, that 84% were drinkers, 44% being binge drinkers. These students spent 5.5 billion on alcohol which was more than they spent on non-alcoholic drinks and text books. Binge drinkers are seven to ten times as likely to have unprotected sex, have trouble with the police, have DUI's, and exhibit violent behavior. Fraternity and sorority students are the most liable to have problems, most likely due to the peer pressure exerted. At age 60, 59% of binge drinkers still abuse alcohol.

Alcohol can be habit forming, create a dependency, destroy family life, destroy careers, create serious health problems, and is responsible for over 100,000 deaths a year in this country. Alcohol interacts with many other drugs, and affects the nervous system, the stomach and the liver. It can have a variety of effects. When intoxicated inhibitions are lowered, some people become belligerent and destructive, others become withdrawn, while a few become "happy drunks." Perhaps this is related to their basic personality. The impaired vision and reaction time is related to numerous accidents, both individual and automobile. In pregnant women, alcohol leads to lower birth weight in children with more health problems, an increase in spontaneous abortion and children with Fetal Alcohol Syndrome which causes severe mental and physical defects. Alcohol can cause degeneration of the liver, called cirrhosis, stomach inflammation, and mental deterioration. Many alcoholics drink at the expense of eating, and the resulting nutritional deficiency contributes to the damages and makes them less able to withstand the toxic effects of the alcohol. The insurance industry feels that alcohol related deaths are under-reported, so there are likely more than the 100,000 deaths. In Colorado, efforts are being made to get drunk drivers off the road in a program called "The Heat is On," *(41)* which was started in 1996. In the succeeding three years, DUI's were up 29%, and alcohol-related accidents were down 23%.

At my alma mater, Southern Methodist University in Dallas, Texas, a 1998 survey found that 78% of students had consumed alcohol in the previous 30 days, 57% of that being binge drinking. Of those, 77% were under the 21 year old legal age for drinking in Texas. One SMU student, badly injured and blinded by a drunken fall, reported that he had started drinking at 14 with a fake ID. Four of five members of fraternities and sororities were binge drinkers. SMU, as are other colleges, is making an active effort to reduce drinking, through stricter enforcement of campus alcohol policy, and a Center for Alcohol and drug abuse. The focus is on education, not punishment. They have also instituted an OCTAA (on the campus talking about alcohol) program. This educational program was done for all their varsity athletes, where drinking is also a problem. This is strange in a group where physical condition is so important. This program teaches, "we don't have any control over our genetic make-up, but we do have control over the choices we make in life." That is exactly what this book is about. SMU also set up a substance-free dorm, and it was the first one to fill up the next semester. Other colleges are taking similar steps to curb the drinking problem.

This does not mean that all drinking is bad. For generations we have kidded about the "medicinal use" of alcohol, and indeed small amounts of alcohol have been found to have beneficial effects. It stimulates gastric secretions to aid digestion, it helps release tensions, and it helps circulation. Alcohol taken at bedtime will relax a person and induce sleep, but it only lasts for two to four hours after which the person wakes up and usually has a hard time going back to sleep. The French have a very low incidence of coronary heart disease which is referred to as "The French Paradox." This was reported in an article in Modern Medicine. *(42)* This is related to the high consumption of wine in France, but the lowered incidence of heart disease did not affect the overall mortality statistics. Dr. William Campbell Douglas reported in his Second Opinion *(43)* that a study done by Dr. Jean-Paul Broustet of Haut Leveque Hospital in France, that red wine contains resveratrol, a substance which increases HDL "good" cholesterol, and limits the artery-blocking LDL cholesterol. I would think that the vasodilating effect of alcohol would also be a factor in dilating the vessels of the heart so clots would be less apt to form and block the vessels. The vasodilating effects of alcohol increase circulation to the skin where the temperature sensors feel the warmth and transmit a message of warmth to the brain, but in cold weather a person is actually losing heat, so drinking can be dangerous when out in the cold. This vasodilating effect is also responsible for many headaches people get from drinking because of congestion in the head, and along with the toxic effects of alcohol is responsible for much of the bad feeling of a hang-over.

There is a story about a fellow who was out drinking with his buddies, and when it came time to go home, he realized that he was in no condition to drive so he called his wife to come and get him. She asked where he was, and he replied that he wasn't sure, but he would go out and look at the street signs. He came back to the phone in a couple of minutes and told his wife, "I'm at the corner of Walk and Don't Walk." The story illustrates that even though the fellow was impaired, at least he had the sense to realize that he needed help to get home. So, take charge of your life and if you drink, do it in moderation.

I will touch only briefly on illicit drugs. Many volumes have been written on the subject, including an outstanding one by

Andrew Weil, M.D. called "The Natural Mind." *(44)* Illicit drugs cause on-going debate and much legislative activity. The bottom line is that these drugs are illegal, because with our present knowledge on the subject, the disadvantages far outweigh any possible benefits. Unfortunately, vast sums of money are involved which leads to crime, and many unnecessary deaths, both from the drugs themselves and from their merchandising.

6

The Environment

There is an old saying that what you don't know won't hurt you. That may be true in some respects, but certainly doesn't apply to our environment. Our environment is polluted by smoke, fumes, dust, hazardous chemicals, radiation, and noise. Many years ago, Albert Schweitzer, M.D., musician, medical missionary, and philosopher made this statement, "Man has lost the capacity to foresee and to forestall. He will end by destroying the earth." The first and most eloquent spokesperson about this problem was Rachel Carson, who compiled a series of articles in the "New Yorker" into her book, "Silent Spring." *(45)* She documented the devastation wrought by the advent of sophisticated pesticides, the first being DDT. That was only the beginning.

Ancient man named four elements - air, earth, water, and fire. We have polluted our air, our earth, and our water, and we use fire frequently to bring about that pollution. We burn hazardous wastes. We use fossil fuels to produce electrical power, as a source of heat in our homes and businesses, and as a source of heat in many manufacturing processes with the production of many toxic chemicals. We burn wood also as a source of heat and the pleasure of watching a fireplace or a bonfire. We accidentally and occasionally start brush and forest fires. We burn carbon fuels in our cars, trucks, buses, farm machines, recreational machines, and many "labor-saving" machines.

Lets start with our air. There is concern over this pollution, the build-up of ozone, the depletion of oxygen, and the "greenhouse" effect. This still appears to be controversial, with vocal proponents on both sides. However, there is no argument about air pollution from internal combustion engines, smoke, dust, and fumes. Los Angeles is notorious for it's air pollution. A few years ago Bob Hope said he had lived in Los Angeles so long that he didn't trust air he couldn't see. A great deal has been done to improve this situation, with fuel additives, more efficient engines, driving restrictions, wood-burning restrictions, etc. In Denver where I live, we for many years were third on the list of most polluted cities, but with concerted efforts to clean up our air, we are no longer in the top ten, showing that progress can be made. This is particularly noteworthy because the population in Denver has increased dramatically in recent years, and continues to do so. The Government has established "acceptable levels" of particulate matter, carbon dioxide, carbon monoxide, and ozone in regard to air pollution.

Another serious problem is the presence of over 80,000 hazardous chemicals which are part of interstate commerce by trucks and railroad tank cars, and always subject to spills and leaks, and the escape of fumes.

Wind kicks up dust which is nearly always more than just dirt. This dust can carry toxic substances, bacteria and viruses. In northern climates, snowy streets are sanded, which after the streets dry out is ground into fine dust, which then is spread into the air. In some areas salt is no longer used as a melting agent, and magnesium chloride has been substituted. There is some question about it's safety, but it leaves a brown film on the windshields, and undoubtedly does the same in lungs.

As bad as our outdoor air is, our indoor air can be even worse, which has been given the name of SBS, the Sick Building Syndrome. Most buildings are now enclosed, and the air is recirculated. It can contain tobacco smoke, construction dust and fumes, other dust especially if carpeted, aerosol sprays, cleaning agents, air "fresheners," polishes, waxes, cosmetics, pet dander, an increasing number of VOC's which are volatile organic compounds, and countless other pollutants. Recent evidence indicates that even some forms of plastic food wrap give off toxic fumes. I believe therefore that there is more and more indication for the use of indoor air filters which combine both particulate and electronic filtration. It has been quite apparent to me from the number of patients who have come home from air travel with respiratory infections, that the recirculated air in airplanes must be a factor in spreading infections. Undoubtedly the change in food and water, and "jet lag" are also factors in lowered resistance to those infections. When travelling, take extra vitamin C, and get some rest.

We are exposed to many forms of radiation, from X-rays, TV sets, microwave ovens, digital clocks, cellular phones, microwave relay antennas, laser pointers, etc. It is advisable not to sit close to TV sets, especially small children. Do not stand close to the microwave oven waiting for food to cook or warm up. Place digital clocks at least 10 feet away from your bed. Do not aim laser pointers at other persons. This has become a popular pastime for the younger generation, but is dangerous.

EMF. There is an electro-magnetic field around every object including the earth. This field is intensified around devices which use electricity, including power lines, transformers, electrical appliances, electric blankets, heating pads, etc. The intensity of EMF decreases as the distance from the source increases. Some levels appear to be harmful. Do not leave electrical appliances on when not being used. If you use an electric blanket in the winter, warm the bed before retiring and then turn it off when you go to bed. Use a hot water bottle instead of a heating pad. Experts tell us that high powered transmission lines don't cause cancer, but the incidence of leukemia is higher in children who live close to transmission lines, and the incidence is higher in adults who work around electric utilities, electrical machinery and welding. When you have a little EMF, some "acceptable" air pollution, some contaminated water, a little pesticide on your vegetables, some coloring agents and preservatives in your food, and a few other things, all of which assault your neuro-muscular system and immune system, it can't help but affect your health eventually.

Another danger is Radon gas. This comes from the breakdown of Radium 226, which in turn comes from the breakdown of Uranium 238. It is prevalent all across the United States, but especially in areas where there are Uranium tailings. This gas can seep into houses and buildings through cracks in the foundations. The National Center for Atmospheric Research lists Radon as a cause of lung cancer, especially if combined with smoking. Richard L Crowther, FAIA, discusses this thoroughly in his book "Indoor Air: Risks and Remedies." *(46)* The Uranium tailings were a product of the atomic age. We are 50 years into the atomic age and have just recently come up with supposedly safe disposal sites for our atomic wastes, but those accumulated wastes have to be transported to the storage sites, one in New Mexico, by truck. The containers are reported to be accident-resistant, but the Titanic was reported to be unsinkable. When our Denver International Airport was being completed, and there was so much trouble with the computerized baggage system, some wag suggested that they put the atomic wastes on that baggage system and they would disappear.

Noise is another type of pollution. Our ears and nervous systems are frequently bombarded by harmful and dangerous levels of noise, such as traffic, jet planes, loud music, sirens, construction, fire arms, thunder, etc. Such noise has been shown to be harmful. Noise levels are measured in decibels. Average city noise runs between 60 - 65 decibels. Possibly hazardous noise is between 80 - 90 decibels and would include construction equipment, diesel trucks, and jet planes overhead. Hazardous noise is between 100 - 120 decibels, and would include motorcycles, snowmobiles, jack hammers, lawn mowers and motor boats. Painful noise is between 120 -130 decibels, and includes very loud music, fire crackers, and jets taking off. Painful and damaging noise is above those levels, and would include firearms, and close sirens.

Food. We have already pointed out that most of our food is deficient in both vitamins and minerals, and much of it is picked "green" so it can be shipped. Many foods also contain coloring agents, preservatives, artificial flavors, artificial sweeteners, and other substances that were not meant to go in our stomachs. Now we are getting genetically altered food in an attempt to increase production. There has not been the opportunity to see what the long-term effects are. An article in U.S. News and World Reports *(47)* lists some of the possible risks. It may enhance some of the plant toxins, but we won't know until people start dieing. It may create new allergies thru altered plant proteins. It may alter the nutrition in unknown ways. It may alter antibiotic resistance. It may upset some environmental balance. And it may spawn some super weeds. In England, some genetic farms have been vandalized. It is estimated that at present somewhere between 25 to 45% of our food is genetically altered, and within 5 years it will be 100%. And now hogs are being genetically treated to alter the smell of their manure, and granted, nothing smells much worse. Their foods are being altered to reduce the smell and chemical content of the manure. This cannot help but alter the composition of the meat.

There are other associated problems with our food. Many fertilizers are artificial and lack natural organic components. According to an article in The Denver Post, *(48)* some manufacturers are using the chemicals from industrial wastes to produce fertilizer, and they contain hazardous chemicals such as lead, cadmium, and arsenic. To make matters worse, each year about a million acres of farm land is being lost to urban sprawl, much of it fertile land which is irreplaceable. Add to that the topsoil which is lost each year due to erosion, and we are losing a great deal. Garbage. We are running out of room to dispose of our wastes. We can no longer dump our wastes in the oceans and rivers and let it wash away. Our landfills are filling up, and many of them are polluting ground water and surrounding soils. We need to do more re-cycling, and find ways to produce energy from our wastes.

Our environment is facing ever-increasing threats. In 1804 the world population was one billion. In 1960 it reached 3 billion. In July of 1999 it reached 6 billion. Every 20 minutes we gain 3,500 persons, but we lose one species of plant or animal, 27,000 per year. We are getting more pollution, we are cutting down more rain forests, losing more farmland, using more water, and creating more hazardous wastes. Where will it end? We need to take the bull by the horns and do something about all these problems. One thing about it, when you have the bull by the horns, you don't have to worry about what is coming out the other end!

Section II

The Structure–Function Relationship of the Human Body

Section II Table of Contents

7

Healing

T he structural integrity of the human body, and it's ability to function normally and efficiently are inexorably intertwined. If the normal structure is altered in any way, either through trauma, stress, posture, disuse or whatever, it will inevitably alter the body's ability to function. Conversely, if the body's function is compromised either through deficiencies, disease, disuse, stress, or whatever, it will also inevitably alter structure, either at the cellular level, or the gross anatomy. As examples of this, cirrhosis of the liver is a cellular change of the liver due to prolonged poisoning from chemicals, often alcohol. The liver becomes enlarged, nodular, and fibrotic, and then can no longer adequately metabolize food. On the gross level, anyone who has had their arm in a cast, which doesn't allow the arm to function, is aware of how quickly the arm muscles become weak and smaller, evidence of structural change.

The human body is truly a miracle. When you stop to think that it starts from one cell which has all the chemical organizers and genes which direct it's division, multiplication, differentiation, and production of trillions of cells, ending with a unique individual unlike any other on earth. Is there a supreme being? I firmly believe so. Part of that Supreme Being's wisdom is to provide every living creature with the ability to overcome injury and disease. We all recognize that injuries heal, but more severe injuries leave permanent impairments because there is a limit to our regenerative powers. Too few recognize that the body is equipped to overcome disease because of it's innate ability to heal, primarily due to the immune system. Proper nutrition is vitally important in this process. However, Medicine continues to tell us to take a pill of some kind for every problem that comes along. This is often not the best answer. Ancient skulls with trephining (holes drilled in the skull) show evidence of healing bone, in spite of the crude instruments that were used, unsterile conditions, and who knows what kind of after care. Ancient writings show many references to healing of many kinds.

The roots of organized medicine which we now recognize, go back to ancient Egypt. They had a caste system of healthcare providers, from bandagers who wrapped the mummies, therapists, physicians and priests. Only priests were allowed to touch the Pharaoh. They worshipped many gods, and used magic, animal products, excrements, and blood. This movement spread to ancient Greece where they did away with the mysticism, superstition, and offensive substances. They started examining the body more closely as the source of problems. Over a period of time two different philosophies arose. The first was the Hippocratic philosophy. This may have been a group of individuals, or one person, Hippocrates, "the father of medicine." He expelled the many gods, and advocated diet, exercise, few drugs, fresh air, mental health, and practiced some form of manipulation. He recognized that environmental factors affect our health. Hippocrates was apparently born on the island of Cos in 460 BC. He had an uncanny power of observation, and advocated gentleness and avoiding harsh measures. He stressed both diagnosis and prognosis. At the same time in another area of Greece called Cnidus the same medical movement from Egypt took a different turn. They confused the diagnosis with the symptoms, then focused on the symptoms, and treated the symptoms. They were not concerned with the prognosis, and insisted on naming every condition. This was the root of the ICDA, the international classification of diseases which doctors spend so much time with today. The Hippocratic philosophy was much more rational, but required more time and effort. The physician had to explain to the patient what the problem was, outline what the patient needed to do, and do what he could do to assure patient compliance. The patient then had to remember the doctors recommendations, and put them into practice. It to some extent recognized the structure-function relationship. The Cnidian philosophy was more simple. The physician focused on the symptoms, gave them a name, and prescribed something to counteract the symptoms, which the patient then needed to take. The Hippocratic philosophy gradually died out and the Cnidian philosophy has persisted to this day, with some exceptions.

Throughout history there have been some who have recognized that the body does attempt to heal and overcome disease. How else would we have survived?

Voltaire 1694 - 1778, the famous, controversial French writer and philosopher said, "the art of medicine is to amuse the patient while nature cures the disease." Voltaire had little respect for doctors, saying, " they poured drugs of which they knew little to cure diseases of which they knew less into human beings of whom they knew nothing." *(49)*

Christian Frederick Hahnemann 1755-1843, a German M.D. was dissatisfied with the practice of medicine, and in 1796 proposed his "Law of Similars." *(50)* He found that by introducing a highly diluted foreign substance into the body which would simulate a certain disease, he could stimulate the body to counter-act that specific disease. Homeopathy gained wide acceptance and spread throughout Europe and the United States. In the United States where many states were attempting to improve medical education, and where new ideas were not readily accepted, as has been the history of Medicine, Homeopathy became branded as quackery, and in the mid 1840's the American Medical Association was formed, primarily to combat the spread of Homeopathy. *(51)*

Ignaz Phillip Semmelweis 1818-1865, *(50)* a Vienna obstetrical assistant where maternity hospitals had a 50% mortality rate, did not feel that the patients were having a fair chance to resist puerperal sepsis and childbed fever, the main causes of the mortalities. Doctors went directly from the dissection lab and morgue to the delivery room without washing their hands. Doctors wore blood and pus covered lab coats to attest to their experience! In portions of the hospital where mid-wives did the deliveries, the mortality rate was less than 20%. Semmelweis advocated washing their hands in chloride of lime. He was ridiculed, driven from Vienna, and died in a lunatic asylum. His ideas were subsequently proven by his students, and by the establishment of Pasteur's germ theory.

Edward Jenner 1749-1823 *(50)* discovered vaccination for small pox, a deadly disease. He had noticed that milk maids who had recovered from cow pox were immune to small pox. He found that by introducing matter from cow pox pustules into a superficial cut on the arm, it created immunity to small pox. He showed that the body's own immune system could be stimulated to be even more resistant to specific diseases.

Louis Pasteur 1822-1895 *(52)* proposed the germ theory, but was ridiculed. He also found that the body could be stimulated to resist disease by introducing a foreign substance, a process he called vaccination. He proved his theory with cholera, anthrax, and later with rabies.

Robert Koch 1843-1910 also found by introducing foreign substances into the body that he could stimulate the body to resist diseases. He developed vaccination for tuberculosis and cholera, and in the process discovered mycobacterium tuberculosis the cause of TB. This opened the field of bacteriology, with many subsequent vaccines produced, proving that the body's own immune system could be enhanced to resist disease.

Ely Metchnikoff 1845-1916 investigated the idea of immunity, and discovered phagocytosis, the process where the body's white blood cells ingest foreign substances. This opened the whole new field of immunology. Metchnikoff shared the Nobel Peace prize in 1908 for his work.

Albert Schweitzer 1875-1965 the famed musician, theologian, philosopher, and missionary doctor, recognized that the results of native witch doctors in Lamborene, Africa, and his own successes in health care were mainly due to the " doctor within," *(52)* referring of course to the body's inherent ability to heal.

In 1910 in her native Australia, Sister Kenny 1886-1952 *(49)*, treated polio with hot packs, passive exercise, and careful physical therapy. This was in direct contrast to the traditional medical treatment of rest and immobilization, and of course she was ridiculed. The rest and immobilization caused atrophy (wasting) of muscles and permanent paralysis, whereas Sister Kenny's hot packs enhanced the body's fever which overcomes the virus, and the motion improved function, enhanced circulation, and promoted healing. In 1933 Sister Kenny opened an institute in Minneapolis to promote her work, which then became unnecessary with the development of polio vaccine in 1953.

Norman Cousins became famous with his book "Anatomy of an Illness as Perceived by the Patient." *(53)* There is a common misconception that he laughed his way out of his illness, but it is much more involved than that as he explains in his book. He suffered a severe debilitating illness in 1969 and was hospitalized. His affliction was recognized as a connective tissue disease and finally diagnosed as "ankylosing spondylitis." Today he would be diagnosed as severe fibromyalgia. Ankylosing spondylitis is a progressive arthritic fusing of the spine, whereas Mr. Cousins problem appears to have been of the soft tissues (muscles, fascias, and ligaments). He was put on large doses of aspirin and an anti-inflammatory, treating the symptoms. This gave him some relief from the pain, but his reading of medical literature told him that both had serious side-effects. He refused to give in to the disease and felt he had a measure of responsibility for his own recovery, feeling that the body does have the ability to recover. This has two-fold importance. First recognizing that the body can heal, and having a positive mental attitude. Further reading told him that vitamin C was important in inflammatory conditions, and that aspirin destroys vitamin C in the body. I would add parenthetically at this point that steroids which are potent anti-inflammatory agents and commonly prescribed in inflammatory conditions, cause excretion of vitamin C, the very substance the body needs to combat the problem! Mr. Cousins also reasoned that if negative thoughts have a negative effect on the body, then positive thoughts ought to have a positive effect. He found that laughter from funny videos and jokes gave him some temporary relief from pain. So he took more control of his destiny and became the "master of his fate, and the captain of his soul." He withdrew from pain medication, started large doses of intravenous vitamin C with his doctor's help, and used humor regularly. He felt that typical hospital routine was not good for ill people with poor food, (see section I chapter 1) interrupted sleep, (see section I chapter 3) unnecessary tests and over-medication (see section I chapter 5), so he moved to a hotel, continued his program and eventually recovered. Some doctors attributed it all to the " placebo effect," but the key things were his positive mental outlook, and the vitamin C which is very important for the connective tissues to heal.

More recently Bernie Siegal, M.D. in "Love, Medicine and Miracles" (54) writes about lessons he has learned about self-healing. He recognizes that the body does heal, and puts some emphasis on the doctor's attitude, but puts most emphasis on the patient's attitude. This is important in promoting healing which we discussed in section I chapter 4, but there is a much more basic and universal mechanism which we will explore later in this section. Dr. Siegel also graphically illustrates the rejection of new ideas by traditional medicine. He relates his experience of putting an item on the bulletin board of his hospital doctor's lounge about the benefits of prayer in reducing post-myocardial infarction complications. Within 24 hours, some doctor had written "B.S." across the report.

Herbert Benson, M.D. *(55)* in his book "Timeless Healing" states, "I've found no healing force more impressive or more universally accessible than the power of the individual to care for and cure him or herself." He explains this by saying that the body remembers what it feels like to be well and comfortable, and then is able to return to that state, relating it to the placebo effect. He diagramed health and well-being as similar to a three-legged stool, the three supports being pharmaceutical, surgery and procedures, and self care. He got off to a good start, but took a wrong turn.

Andrew Weil, M.D. *(56)*, author of "Spontaneous Healing" understands that the body has the ability to heal, but frankly admits he can't explain how. He states in his book, "The survival of the species alone implies the existence of a healing system." He goes on to say, "My purpose in writing this book is to convince more people to rely on the body's innate potential for maintaining health and overcoming illness, but I cannot easily give you a picture of the system." I admire Dr. Weil a great deal. He has made a significant contribution to holistic health care through his writing, his teaching, and his health center in Tucson. He is a broad-minded, free-thinking physician who has escaped from the Cnidian brainwashing doctors get in medical school which is so much a part of "traditional" medicine.

Andrew Taylor Sill, M.D. We must go back to the 19th century to find the physician who fully understood the body's inherent ability to heal, was able to describe it, and developed a system of healing which most completely promotes the body's response to it's fullest potential. Dr. Still practiced at the time of the Civil War. As with some of the previous medical pioneers we have discussed, he too was dissatisfied with the practice of medicine, and admittedly it was crude at that time. After some extended deliberation, and some agonizing experiences, he developed a philosophy which he hoped would improve the practice of medicine, surgery, and obstetrics. As with many other medical pioneers, his ideas were rejected, he was ridiculed, and so he established a new school of medicine which he called Osteopathy. We shall examine Dr. Still and his philosophy in the next chapter.

8

A. T. Still – the Formative Years

Andrew Taylor Still was born August 6th, 1828 in Jonesboro, Lee County, Virginia. The log cabin he was born in is now safely under cover at the Kirksville College of Osteopathic Medicine in Kirksville, Missouri. Jonesboro was on Boone's Wilderness Road, a major east-west thoroughfare. His parents were Abram Still, M.D. and Martha Poage Moore Still. Dr. Abram Still was a Methodist Episcopal circuit rider, ministering to both the medical and spiritual needs of the people. He was also a farmer. He expected his children to help with the farming, and he frequently took them along when he was treating the sick. In 1834 the Stills moved to New Market, Tennessee, still on the Wilderness Road. Then in 1836 they moved to Macon county, Missouri, which was on a north-south thoroughfare of it's day. There had been some threats on the life of the Doctor Reverend Still because of his very strong anti-slavery views, so the church Elders transferred him as a safety precaution.

Being raised on these major thoroughfares exposed Andrew, or Drew as he was called as a child, to many people, sources of information, and many new ideas. Drew was an inquisitive child, and a thinker. On November 13, 1833 when he was five, there was a spectacular display of falling stars. Some adults thought it portended the end of the world, but Drew asked, "what made that happen?" When he was about ten he was suffering from headaches. He strung a plow rope a few inches above the ground between two trees, laid a blanket over it and then lay down with his neck on the padded rope and found that it relieved his headache. He used this method for many years and finally realized when he was older and more aware of anatomy that this was relieving muscle tension in his neck, and improving blood and nerve supply, and thereby easing his headaches. It was some 120 years later that some portions of the medical profession began to understand the relationship of neck tension and some types of headache.

Growing up on the frontier, Andrew observed the works of nature, was deeply religious because of his father's influence, and with his hunting and cleaning game had learned a good deal about anatomy. He was beginning to take an interest in his father's medical practice. One day as a boy, he was sitting at the edge of a field reading one of his father's medical books. His father said, "Drew, I told you not to read my books in the field," whereupon Drew turned around, put his feet in the road and kept on reading.

In 1840 the Stills moved to Schyler county, Missouri, and then in 1844 close to the present day Macon, Missouri, again on a north-south thoroughfare. In 1849, Andrew, now a strapping young man, married Mary Vaughn. In 1853 they moved to Wakarusa Mission, Kansas where Dr. Abram Still was missionary to the Shawnee Indians. This was on the Santa Fe Trail and during the California gold rush, with a great deal of westward travel. Andrew was serving a medical preceptorship with his father which was customary in those days. He later attended a Medical School in Baldwin, Kansas. In 1857 he was elected to the Kansas Legislature as a free state candidate. In 1859 his wife Mary died of cholera, which was epidemic among the Indians they were serving. Then in 1860 he married Mary E. Turner, the daughter of a doctor. She proved to be a staunch and faithful supporter through the trying years which were to follow.

In 1861 Dr. Still enlisted in the 9th Kansas Cavalry at Fort Leavenworth. For many years emotions had been running high over the slavery issue, and Dr. Still was a strong abolitionist. There had been bush-whacking, shooting, burning, and a great deal of violence. Dr. Still had been in many dangerous situations, but his bravery and skill as a doctor created respect from his adversaries, and he was allowed to make his rounds as a doctor. In 1862 his cavalry unit was disbanded, but Dr. Still organized a unit of Kansas Militia, and patrolled the Santa Fe Trail. In 1864 a major battle was fought on the Kansas-Missouri border, during which several musket balls passed through Dr. Still's clothing. Having routed the pro-slavery forces, Dr. Still, then a major, received orders to disband. He drew his regiment up in line, told them they had a long march ahead of them, but that no one would be forced to go. He asked for volunteers, about one third stepped forward. He then read the order to disband, dismissed them, and sent them home, as related in his autobiography. *(57)*

Dr. Still had experienced a growing dissatisfaction with the practice of Medicine. This was reinforced by a surgeon friend of his in the army who had voiced similar dissatisfaction. Dr. Still was particularly concerned by the prevalence of low back pain and wondered what anatomic problems caused it. He was disturbed by the frequent use of morphine to control back pain and the number of patients who became addicted to it. He started experimenting with manual methods to relieve back pain, and found it was helpful in many cases.

During the Civil War all doctors had been taken into the service and when Dr. Still returned home it was quite apparent that fewer children had died when the doctors were away. This seemed strange at the time, but under investigation is not strange at all. Their favorite medicine was Calomel, which is chloride of mercury, a deadly poison. They also used sulfuric acid and salt, corrosive sublimate or bichloride of mercury, sugar (acetate) of lead, strychnine, poison oak, and potassium cyanide *(58), (59)*. Their "medicines" were actually killing their patients! Have things changed much with over 160,000 persons a year now dying from drug reactions? In Dr. Still's time they also used a number of herbs which are still in use such as cayenne pepper, fox glove (digitalis), ginseng, and golden seal. Modern research has proven the beneficial effects of many herbs.

Then tragedy struck. The Still family had come through the war unscathed, but an epidemic of spinal meningitis claimed three of Dr. Still's children. He watched in horror as they got sicker and sicker, their fevers kept climbing, their pain got worse, and they were begging him to do something. Then one by one they suffered convulsions, coma and death. He and his medical colleagues were powerless to do anything. So as stated in his autobiography *(57)*, "In sickness has God left man in a world of guessing? Guess what is the matter? What to give, and guess the result? And dead, guess where he goes? I decided then that God is not a guessing God, but a God of truth. And all his works, spiritual and material are harmonious. His love of animal life is absolute. So wise a God had certainly placed the remedy within the material house in which the spirit of life dwells. Believing that a loving intelligent maker of man had deposited in his body in some place or throughout the whole system, drugs in abundance to cure all infirmities, that all the remedies necessary to health exist in the human body." This demonstrates a tremendous faith in his creator. With this belief firmly in mind, and with this steadfast faith, he set out to find his answers. He prayed for guidance, and he studied human anatomy in greater detail. He dissected many bodies, using Indian bodies as his subjects. A number of books have portrayed Dr. Still as a grave robber, but his grandson, Charles E. Still, Jr. in his book "Frontier Doctor, Medical Pioneer" *(59)* paints a much different picture. An epidemic of cholera had killed hundreds of Indians, because they had no immunity to it, and there had been mass burials. The Indians had been moved to several reservations, so their burial grounds were no longer sacred places. Dr. Still and his father had been medical missionaries to the Indians for many years, so they knew him well. Their Chief gave Dr. Still permission to exhume bodies, which was of great benefit in learning anatomy in greater detail. Then he started examining his patients more carefully looking for physical causes for their complaints and illnesses. It must be remembered that Dr. Still did have crude surgical instruments, (his wartime surgical kit is in the Smithsonian Institute), but he had no diagnostic instruments, no laboratories, no reference books, nothing but his special senses, his keen intellect, an inquiring mind, and a burning desire to find the truth. He said in his autobiography *(57)*, "that one's brain is his only reliable friend." He paid particular attention to the blood and nerve supply of the body and concluded that all diseases are effects of dysfunction of those important systems. He stated in his autobiography *(57)* "The cause can be found and does exist in the limited or excited action of the nerves which control the fluids of part or the whole of the body." This was a very profound conclusion showing he was understanding the function of the autonomic nervous system, which was the object of some experiments in Europe in the late 1800's, but was not named until 1898 by Langley, and was not accurately described until the early 1900's. *(60)*

In addition to this was the first of many conclusions Dr. Still reached about how the human body functions, the causes of disease, and the body's inherent ability to heal, all of which have been proven by modern research. He was convinced that his philosophy was the truth he had been seeking, that his methods were correct, and that it would be of great benefit to mankind. So on June 22, 1874 he "flung to the breeze the banner of Osteopathy." *(57)*

In addition to his complete, detailed knowledge of anatomy which he always stressed to his students, Dr. Still had an uncanny understanding of the function of the human body. As has been said before, this was entirely without the aid of laboratory tests, instruments of any kind, or imaging from X-rays, scans or MRI's, which are so commonly done today. In 1898 Dr. Still installed an X-ray machine in his infirmary, which was the second one west of the Mississippi. This was only two years after Wilhelm Roentgen discovered X-ray. *(61)*

Dr. Still had reached many of his conclusions through his study of anatomy, having said, "begin and end with anatomy" *(62)*, and with his powers of reasoning. He stated, "the student of any philosophy succeeds best by the more simple methods of reasoning." "The explorer for truth must first declare his independence of all obligations or brotherhoods of any kind what-so-ever. He must be free to think and reason." *(ibid)* "The Osteopath reasons, if he reasons at all, that order and health are inseparable, that when order in all parts is found, disease cannot prevail." *(ibid)*

His understanding of human physiology is illustrated by the following. "If we think as men of reason should, we will count five nerve powers. They must all be present to build a part, and must answer promptly to roll call and work all the time. The names of these master workmen are sensation, motions, nutrition, voluntary and involuntary." *(ibid)* This was a very profound statement at a time when actual knowledge of the formation and function of the nervous system was very meager. The human nervous system is made up of two major divisions, the voluntary and the involuntary. Both of these have two sub-divisions. The voluntary nervous system has the sensory division which gives us pain, touch and temperature, and the motor division which gives us voluntary control of muscles. The involuntary nervous system is made up of the sympathetic portion which is spoken of as the "fright or flight" mechanism. It controls circulation and also provides the expenditure of energy in fear, temperature changes, emotional outbursts, physical activity and pain. It also contributes to many chronic pain syndromes. The para-sympathetic nervous system on the other hand promotes homeostasis and basic bodily functions. The fact that the nervous system has a nutritional function was proven by I. M. Korr, Ph. D. in 1981. This will be discussed in Chapter ten. Dr. Still went on to say, "Is he (the D.O.) not justified in the conclusion that the nerves do gestate and send forth all substances that are applied by nature in it's construction of man?" *(ibid)*

In 1874, the year Dr. Still proclaimed Osteopathy, he said, "a disturbed artery marked the beginning to an hour and a minute when disease began to sow it's seeds of destruction in the human body. The rule of the artery must be absolute, universal and unobstructed, or disease will be the result." *(57)* Some years later he elaborated on that in his "Philosophy of Osteopathy" with these statements. "The Osteopath sees the various parts of this great system (the circulatory system) of life when preparing fluids commonly known as blood, passing through a set of tubes both great and small, some so vastly small as to require the aid of powerful microscopes to see their infinitely small forms, through which the blood and other fluids are conducted by the heart and force of the brain, to construct organs, muscles, membranes, and all the things necessary to life and motion, to the parts separately and combined." "Blood, an unknown fluid. It is in all parts of flesh and bone. When Harvey [William Harvey, 1578-1657, a British Physician who first described circulation] *(49)* solved by his power of reason a knowledge of the circulation of blood, he only reached the banks of the river of life. He saw that the heads and mouths of the rivers of blood begin and end in the heart, to do the mysterious works of constructing man. Blood is systematically funneled from the heart to all divisions of our bodies. The rule of the artery and vein is universal in all living beings, and the Osteopath must know that, and abide by it's rulings, or he will not succeed as a healer." (62)

In saying, "Pure and healthy blood, the greatest known germicide," he recognized the bodies ability to overcome disease, which we now know is due to our immune system with the distribution of white blood cells and anti-bodies by adequate circulation. Dr. Still showed further insight into the body's inherent immunity when he said, "I know of no part of the body that equals the fascia as a hunting ground for disease." "Fascia, it being that principle that sheaths, permeates, divides and sub-divides every portion of all animal bodies. By it's action we live, and by it's failure we shrink, or swell, or die. This life is surely too short to solve the uses of fascia in animal forms." *(ibid)* Today we know that fascia contains significant elements of what is commonly known as the reticulo-endothelial system, with both fixed and mobile cells which destroy invading pathogenic agents, whether they be viruses, bacteria, fungi, parasites, or allergic agents. This system would be better known as the Monocyte-macrophage System. *(15)*

Dr. Still also said, "fever is a natural and powerful remedy." *(62)* The fever is part of increased metabolism which enhances the immune system, and the increased temperature helps eliminate pathogens, particularly viruses. This is why Sister Kenney's hot pack treatment was effective against polio. Too many of today's doctors consider a fever just a symptom and prescribe an anti-pyretic (to lower fever) such as aspirin or tylenol. This interferes with the body's natural response to an infection. It is no wonder people who are treated that way so often stay sick so long.

Dr. Still understood the importance of the cerebro-spinal fluid in it's relationship to the health of the brain. He called the cerebro-spinal fluid "the highest known element that is contained in the human body, and unless the brain formulates this fluid in abundance a disabled condition of the body will remain. He who is able to reason will see that this great river of life must be tapped and the withering field irrigated at once, or the harvest of health is forever lost." *(67)* This expanding concept, Cranio-sacral Osteopathy, was developed by an early student of Dr. Still's, William Garner Sutherland, and we will discuss it in chapter 12. Dr. Still did not have to deal with the refined foods we have today, which deprive us of adequate nutrition, but he understood the importance bio-chemistry. He said, "Then chemistry is of great use as a part of a thorough Osteopathic education. It gives us reason why food is found in the body as bone, muscle, and so on, to all kinds of flesh, teeth and bone found in animal forms. Osteopathy believes that all parts of the human body do work on chemical compounds, and from the general supply manufacture for local wants." *(ibid)* He referred to the liver as "natures chemical laboratory." We know today that our food is metabolized in the liver, and those metabolic products are utilized in every cell by additional chemical reactions.

Dr. Still's deep religious beliefs, and the importance of the spiritual aspect of healing is exemplified by his body-mind-spirit concept, saying, "first the material body, second the spiritual being, and third a being of mind which is far superior to all vital motions and material forms, whose duty is to wisely manage the great engines of life." *(ibid)* He often referred to God as the "Master Mechanic."

Dr. Still expected much of his students. He required that they make a grade of 95 in order to pass anatomy. He expected his students to recognize and understand the truths he was teaching them when he said, "No one truth is greater than any other truth. Treat with respect and reverence all truths." *(ibid)* "To the Osteopath his first and last duty is to look to a healthy blood and nerve supply." *(ibid)* "To find health should be the object of the doctor, anyone can find disease." And he said, "An Osteopath should be a clear-headed, conscientious, truth-loving man, and never speak until he knows he has found and can demonstrate the truth he claims to know." *(ibid)*

Dr. Still dealt with the doctor-patient relationship when he said, "People expect more than guessing from an Osteopath." *(ibid)* A true Osteopath has special palpatory skills which allows him or her to do a thorough physical diagnosis, a lost art with much of the medical profession. A careful examination of the tissues - the skin, fascia, muscles, ligaments, and bone will reveal a great deal of information about that patient, and does away with much of the guess-work which then requires the frequent X-rays, MRI's, ultra-sound, and numerous laboratory tests. The imaging and lab tests are then minimized to confirm a diagnosis, or rule out certain other things. We will go into this in detail in chapter 13.

9

Establishing the Osteopathic Profession

D r. Still did not set out to establish a new school of medicine. His idea was "to improve the practice of medicine, surgery and obstetrics." *(57)* However, he had great difficulty in getting his ideas accepted. Most of his medical colleagues rejected his ideas, as had happened to Semmelweis, Hahnemann, Koch, Jenner, Pasteur, and even Sister Kenny. As Booth stated in his "History of Osteopathy," *(60)* "No great discovery was ever made by one who stuck to the paths already established." Preachers denounced Dr. Still, some of the public ridiculed him, even some of his own family thought he was crazy. He was convinced his ideas were correct because he was getting results with his manipulation. He felt his ideas and methods needed more exposure so he asked to present his concept at Baldwin University which he and his brother had founded by donating land and helping with the construction. The doors were closed to him which was a bitter disappointment. The general mood of the people may have been a factor because there was a financial panic in the East at that time, and there was a severe locust plague on the frontier at the same time.

Dr. Still's new manipulation methods were getting results,

but many of the people who asked for his help would ask him to come by the back door, or come at night so they wouldn't be seen consulting with him.

In 1875 Dr. Still moved to Kirksville, Missouri and soon proved himself by helping some difficult cases. One of the first was a Mrs. Harris. She had been sick for years, and all of the M.D.'s in town had given up on her. She was not able to raise her head, was subject to cramps and convulsions, was often unconscious, and vomited almost constantly. Dr. Still treated her for about three months, after which she enjoyed good health for many years. *(60)* During this time he travelled to other towns, both to spread the word about Osteopathy and to see more ailing patients. Another case which demonstrates both his ability and his benevolent nature occurred in the company of a Dr. Patterson, who took over the management of Dr. Still's financial affairs. They met an old colored lady with a crooked neck and a spasm in the muscles. Dr. Still placed one foot on the second plank of a fence, and with the old lady resting against his knee, placed one hand on her neck, the other on her head, and gave it a twist that corrected the problem at once. The old lady, quite happy, asked him his price. Dr. Still asked, "what is your name and what do you do?" Finding she was a poor washerwoman, he said, "that will be ten dollars." Her purse was empty so she replied, "All right Massa, but I has to get some clothes to wash before I kin pay you." Dr. Still put his hand in his pocket, pulled out a ten dollar bill, gave it to her, and said, "your bill is paid, go home and be happy." It was such good work and generosity that attracted much attention to Dr. Still. It also got him the nick-name of "the lightening bone-setter." *(60)*

In later years Dr. Still said to his pupils, "No preacher will pray for you as one possessed of a devil, no innocent children will fly from your presence in fear of one spoken of as a lunatic. No, your fate will not be my fate, for my untiring efforts placed this science and it's exponents upon a footing to command the respect and admiration of the world." *(57)*

Within a few years his fame had spread, and patients were coming to Kirksville from all over the world. The Wabash railroad had to put extra trains on their line to Kirksville from St. Louis to handle the crowds of people seeking his services. Among the notables he treated during that time were Helen Keller and Samuel Clemmons (Mark Twain).

Dr. Still's understanding of anatomy and the function of the human body was astounding. His knowledge and his military background are illustrated in this statement from his autobiography. "Every corpuscle goes like a man in the army, with full instructions where to go, and with unerring precision it does it's work - whether it be in the formation of a hair or the throwing of a spot of delicate tinting at certain distances on a peacock's back." *(57)* Dr. J.H. Sullivan, an M.D. who brought his wife to Dr. Still for treatment said, "In anatomy, vast as the subject is and as intricate as well, Dr. Still has within him an almost supernatural acquaintance with the living model." *(60)*

By the late 1880's Dr. Still was unable to handle the crowds that were seeking his services, although he had trained his sons Charles, Harry, Herman, and Fred to do some of the work, but he realized that they needed more formal training. Others were asking to learn his methods so as early as 1889 he started thinking about opening a school. In 1891 an informal class was started to train as assistants. *(61)* A charter was applied for and granted by the State of Missouri on May 10, 1892. In June of 1892, Dr. Still was sought out by a William Smith, M.D., from Scotland, a licentiate of the Royal College of Physicians and Surgeons of Edinburgh. Dr. Smith was in Missouri selling medical books and supplies, and he had heard complaints of many M.D.'s about this "quack" who was hurting their business. Dr. Smith spent many hours talking to Dr. Still, thought his theory made a lot of sense, and that same evening agreed to teach anatomy at a new school. Dr. Still was urged to name the school after himself, but he was both patriotic and wanting to benefit all of mankind, so he named it "The American School of Osteopathy." *(61)* The first class was started on October 3, 1992 with eleven students, although there are some contradictions about the exact date. *(61)* Several students were added, and a year later a class of 18 was graduated, which included five women. The second class started in the fall of 1893 with an enrollment of 24 students. Dr. Smith had moved to Kansas City to go into practice, so Dr. Still asked Dr. Jeanette Bolles to teach anatomy. Dr. Bowles was from Denver, had been a member of the first class, and was the first woman Osteopath based on her alphabetical graduation. Dr. Still was always a strong supporter of women. He campaigned vigorously for Women's Suffrage.

History shows that in 1893 D.D. Palmer, a "magnetic healer" from Davenport, Iowa spent two weeks in Kirksville, was treated by Dr. Still and several faculty members, then returned to Davenport and announced his discovery of chiropractic. This is recounted by Arthur Hildreth, D.O., a graduate of the first class and a close friend of Dr. Still's in his book, " The Lengthening Shadow of Andrew Taylor Still," *(63)* by Georgia Walters, the historian of Kirksville in her book, "The First School of Osteopathic Medicine," *(61)* by Dr. Still's grandson Charles Still Jr., D.O. in his book, "Frontier Doctor, Medical Pioneer," *(59)* and referred to briefly by a former chiropractic instructor Mark Sanders, D.C. in an article "Take it From a D.C.: a Lot of Chiropractic is a Sham" which appeared in Medical Economics September 17, 1990 *(64)*

In 1894, the Osteopathic course was increased to two years, and an infirmary was being built. Many of the early graduates moved to other areas and opened their own Osteopathic Colleges. One opened in Kansas City in 1895, in Los Angeles in 1896, in Denver in 1897 by Dr. Bolles, in Massachusetts and Des Moines in 1898, in Philadelphia in 1899, and Chicago in 1900. The Bolles College was combined with the American School of Osteopathy in 1904. Some of the other schools closed, but a few survived. Classes kept increasing in size at Kirksville and new buildings were added, In 1897 a large addition was put on the Infirmary Building. By 1900 classes had grown to over 200 students. During these years Osteopathy had started it's world wide spread. It was introduced to Hawaii in 1897, Canada in 1898, the Philippines in 1899, and soon in Mexico, Ireland, England, China, and the West Indies. *(60)*

Osteopathy was proving itself in many ways. In 1895, a student at the American School of Osteopathy was treating a prominent clothing manufacturer from St. Louis, and accompanied him to his summer home in Vermont to continue treatment. While there he was asked to treat other people and was getting excellent results, including curing the son of a prominent politician of asthma. As word spread, the local M.D.'s rose in complaint, saying an unlicensed person was treating "weak-minded" persons. The weak minded persons turned out to be some of the most prominent people, who rallied in support of Osteopathy. When the M.D.'s sponsored a bill in the legislature to exclude Osteopathy, it was defeated, and a bill to legalize Osteopathy was quickly passed. It was signed by the Governor in November 1996, and thus Vermont became the first state to recognize Osteopathy. Missouri's first attempt for licensure failed in 1895, but passed in 1897. Many early graduates were aware of the importance of legal recognition for their fledgling profession and worked hard to achieve it. An outstanding example of this was David L. Clark, D.O., an early patient of Dr. Still's. As a young man in Iowa, David Clark had fallen out of a tree and broken his back and his pelvis. He had been a cripple for three years when he heard of a Dr. Still in Missouri who was doing some marvelous things. David went to Kirksville and was cured by Dr. Still. He was so impressed he decided to make Osteopathy his own life's work. While carrying the proceeds from selling some property, he was waylaid and beaten by robbers, and left unconscious. He suffered severe headaches but announced his decision to study Osteopathy. Officials ruled him insane and had him incarcerated for a year. When he was released he went to Kirksville again, was again cured by Dr. Still, enrolled, and graduated in 1898. He then went to Texas, the first Osteopath in the state, and became very successful. The medical profession tried to drive him out, but he introduced himself to legislators, told them about Osteopathy, and got practice rights in 1907. He then moved to Colorado where he had worked on the railroad as a young man. He took a room at the Argonaut Hotel, which is still across the street from the Capitol Building, again introduced himself to legislators, treated them and got Colorado's practice law in 1913. *(63)*

Educational requirements were being increased during this time. In 1905 the curriculum at A.S.O. was increased to 3 years, and then to 4 years in 1915. A national organization had been formed in Kirksville in 1897 called the American Association for the Advancement of Osteopathy. The name was changed to the American Osteopathic Association in 1901.

In 1912 on his way to the Convention of the American Osteopathic Association in Denver, Dr. Still was injured in a train wreck. His health was never quite as good after that. Dr. Still died of a stroke at 3:30 P.M. December 17, 1917 at the age of 89. As word got out, telegrams poured in to Kirksville from all over the world. On the afternoon of his funeral service, presided over by his good friend, Dr. Arthur Hildreth, all of the businesses and schools in Kirksville were closed in honor of Dr. Still. Thousands of people gathered in Kirksville for the service. By this time Osteopathy was well established. There were 5,000 Osteopathic Physicians, and six Osteopathic Colleges. They were the American School of Osteopathy, now the Kirksville College of Osteopathic Medicine, the Kansas City College of Osteopathy, now the University of Health Sciences College of Osteopathic Medicine, the Pacific College of Osteopathy taken over by the medical profession in 1962, the Des Moines Still College, now the University of Osteopathic Medicine and Health Sciences / College of Osteopathic Medicine and Surgery, the Chicago College of Osteopathy, now the Chicago College of Osteopathic Medicine Midwestern University, and the Philadelphia College of Osteopathy, now the Philadelphia College of Osteopathic Medicine. At that time nine states had been granted unrestricted practice rights (medicine, surgery, and obstetrics, plus manipulation), many states had practice rights restricted to just manipulation, and a few states had no practice laws, so in many instances Osteopaths were arrested, but always their patients rallied in their support. Osteopaths tended to settle in states where they had unrestricted practice rights, so this created very irregular distribution of Osteopaths. The profession had made significant growth, but there were many challenges ahead.

10

The Growth of the Osteopathic Profession

O steopathy continued to grow and gain wider acceptance after the establishment of other early schools, the formation of organizations to provide unity, the agreement to meet certain basic standards, and the growing clinical success of Osteopathy.

For many years, in spite of Osteopathy's great success and acceptance, the medical profession voiced the constant criticism, "there is no scientific proof." This has been leveled at many other aspects of health care as well. There had been some animal research done to substantiate the Osteopathic concept as early as 1898-99. Then in the early 1900's, Dr. Louisa Burns, a 1903 graduate of the Pacific College of Osteopathy in Los Angeles, launched a significant program of research. A very important part of the Osteopathic concept is the alteration of the internal glands and organs by the interference of blood and nerve supply. Dr. Burns used laboratory animals, usually rabbits, which reproduce quickly and are easily handled. She would gently produce Osteopathic "lesions," now referred to as "somatic dysfunctions," in specific areas of the spine of part of a litter of rabbits with nerve supply related to whatever organ she wished to study. She would leave half of the litter normal as controls. After a certain period of time, she would sacrifice the animals, do histologic examination of their tissues, and document her findings. She published four volumes *(66)* of those findings, and made a significant contribution to Osteopathic literature. She is honored annually by The Bureau of Osteopathic Research with a memorial address. In the early 1940's, J. Stedman Denslow, D. O., a 1929 graduate of the Kirksville College of Osteopathy and Surgery, started a research program using human subjects. This was limited because you don't sacrifice human subjects, but he added additional information on how the human neuro-musculo-skeletal system works, and how it is altered by changes in structure. An article of Dr. Denslow's was published in the Journal of Neuro-physiology in 1941 *(67)*, the first article to be published in a non-Osteopathic scientific journal.

In 1945 Kirksville hired I. M. Korr, Ph.D. to set up a formal research program, and to teach physiology to the Osteopathic students. During the war, Dr. Korr had been doing research for the War Department. In the ensuing years, Dr. Korr and associates such as Elliot Hix and Price Thomas provided very substantial proof of the Osteopathic concept, and made some significant contributions to the field of neuro-physiology. One significant finding was that axons, the nerve filament that conducts nerve impulses away from the nerve cell, have an important function in carrying nutrient substances. *(68)* Before the turn of the century, Dr. Still had noted the nutrient function of nerves. Dr. Korr had planned on staying in Kirksville for only one year to set up the research program, but he became quite interested in the Osteopathic concept and devoted his life to Osteopathic research, many years at Kirksville, later at the Michigan State College of Osteopathic Medicine, and later still at the Texas College of Osteopathic Medicine. Dr. Korr came from a family who had all died in their 40's and 50's, and he had resigned himself to the same fate, but when he got to Kirksville, one of the Osteopathic staff members started treating Dr. Korr regularly and corrected his diet. On August 24, 2000 Dr. Korr celebrated his 91st birthday. Over the years, as an internationally known speaker, Dr. Korr has had much to say about longevity, and Osteopathy's contribution to it. Dr. Korr is retired in Boulder, Colorado, a short distance from Denver. He was my physiology professor in 1946. I have been on many programs with him over the years, both in this country, in Canada, and in Germany. I have the privilege of carrying on Dr. Korr's Osteopathic care since he moved to Boulder.

Many early Osteopathic cases were chronic problems requiring institutional care, so in addition to Osteopathic Hospitals, many Sanatoriums were established which were quite successful. Then in 1950 there was a major breakthrough. In Adrian County Missouri, a court ruled that Osteopathic Physicians (D.O.) have the right to practice in tax supported hospitals. (69) Gradually other hospitals admitted D.O.'s, and now days nearly all hospitals have a joint staff of both M.D.'s and D.O.'s.

Early Osteopathic Physicians (D.O.'s) all did Osteopathic Manipulative Treatment (OMT), including the specialists, whether they were surgeons, obstetricians, psychiatrists, internists or whatever. They got better results because they were helping the body's inherent ability to heal, with whatever else they were doing as a part of their specialty. Non-specialized D.O.'s were doing "general practice," which we now call family practice, and treating all sorts of illness, which again aided the body's own efforts. Others specialized in manipulation (OMT), some by choice, some because their State had not yet granted full practice rights. There have always been some who failed to recognize the great gift Dr. Still gave them, and have just practiced medicine. They have really missed the boat, and undoubtedly there are many reasons for this, but as one of our all-time great Osteopaths, Paul Kimberly, D.O., F.A.A.O. observed years ago, "they tried so hard to show they were as good as M.D's, they became the same as."

Joint staff hospitals have been a mixed blessing. While it is good to have the cooperation and interaction of the two professions, it is good to have the M.D.'s see that Osteopathic Physicians can practice good medicine, and it is good for the M.D.'s to see that Osteopathic Manipulation has much to offer, but not enough of Osteopathic Physicians use manipulation in the hospital setting. And some Osteopathic Physicians do not use OMT in their offices. This has lead some people to think that the use of manipulation in the Osteopathic Profession was on the decline. This was true back in the 50's and 60's when less emphasis was placed on OMT. Some chiropractors said we were giving up manipulation (wishful thinking), and that it was an elective in our colleges, but that is not true. With the addition of 13 new Osteopathic Colleges, and greater emphasis being put on teaching our graduates the art of OMT, the utilization is increasing. Surveys vary, but it is apparent that the majority of D.O.'s do use some OMT. As a general rule, the more you use it, the more proficient one becomes at using it.

Osteopathic Manipulation has survived in spite of many hardships. The early rejection of Dr. Still's ideas was a difficult time, then after the public's enthusiastic reception of Osteopathy it was labeled a "cult" by the Medical Profession, then the American Medical Association tried to absorb the Osteopathic Profession. I related in Chapter 7 of this Section that the AMA was formed to combat the spread of Homeopathy from Germany. Then there was another group of M.D.'s called Eclectics who focused on just one symptom, unlike the Allopaths (todays M.D.'s) who focus on and treat multiple symptoms. The eclectics were absorbed by the Allopaths. Then in 1962 the Medical Profession was successful in getting a referendum passed in California to prohibit the granting of any more Osteopathic licenses in California, and they took over the Los Angeles Osteopathic College. They offered all of the Osteopaths in California the M.D. degree, which about three fourths of the profession accepted. It then became known as the "little M.D. degree," because the D.O.'s that took it lost many of their practice rights. The Medical Association had plans to do this in 16 other states where there was either an Osteopathic College, or a large population of Osteopathic Physicians. Alerted by the catastrophe in California, the other states and the American Osteopathic Association successfully resisted the move. The D.O.'s in California who retained their identity, went to Court and on the basis that patients were being denied their choice of physicians were successful in getting the California Supreme Court to void the 1962 court decision. By this time there was full licensure in all 50 States.

Another significant development in the growth and acceptance of Osteopathy relates to the armed forces medical corps. In World War II many Osteopathic Physicians served in the armed forces, but not in a medical capacity. They were foot soldiers, pilots, sea bees, sailors, etc. However, some were deferred because of the shortage of doctors on the home front. Many M.D.'s, when they returned home from service, were unhappy with the Medical Profession's refusal to let D.O.'s serve in the armed forces medical services, because many of their patients stayed with the Osteopaths who had cared for them during the war. In 1966 D.O.'s were finally authorized to serve in the medical corps of the Army, Navy, and Air Force. In Viet Nam and Desert Storm the D.O.'s were found to better handle a variety of problems. This was because their Osteopathic training gave them a better opportunity to recognize a greater variety of problems and how to deal with them. At the present time more than 20% of the armed forces medical officers are D.O.'s, and many of them have achieved high ranks. Osteopathic Physicians have also come to play a larger role in Public Health and Governmental Health Agencies.

In 1969 another big step in the expansion of the Osteopathic Profession took place. The first new Osteopathic College in several decades was opened at Michigan State University, the Michigan State University College of Osteopathic Medicine. This was in addition to a Medical School and a school of Veterinary Medicine. In that time period where Medical Schools were cutting back because of a "surplus of doctors," other new Osteopathic Colleges were added, and existing Colleges expanded their facilities and enlarged their classes because of the increasing demand for Osteopathic services. As of the year 2000, there are now 45,000 Osteopathic Physicians and 19 Osteopathic Colleges, some of them associated with State Universities, others independently financed. The first Osteopathic College, The Kirksville College of Osteopathic Medicine, had gone through some trying financial times, but elected to stay independent. All Osteopathic Colleges have to meet certain basic requirements established by the American Osteopathic Association, but State supported Colleges also have dictates from State Legislatures. In recent years the Kirksville College of Osteopathic Medicine has built up an enviable endowment fund from it's loyal alumni and from grateful patients of those alumni. I received my pre-medical training in the Navy V-12 program, a concentrated officer procurement program during the Second World War. Many of my Navy friends went to some of the best Medical Schools in the United States, recognized as the best in the world. Having taken State Board exams with some of them, having had extensive teaching experience here and abroad, and having done a great deal of reading of all kinds over the years, there is no doubt in my mind that the Kirksville College of Osteopathic Medicine is the best Health Care teaching institution in the world.

There are two organizations which have contributed significantly to the growth of the Osteopathic Profession, and to the preservation of Dr. Still's principles. The first is the American Academy of Osteopathy. It was started in 1937 at the Convention of the American Osteopathic Association (AOA) in Chicago. A group of 66 prominent Osteopaths, concerned about preserving Dr. Still's teachings met and formed an organization called "The Osteopathic Manipulation and Clinical Research Association." The next year in Cincinnati they were given time on the AOA

Program to make a presentation, which has continued every year. In 1941 the name was changed to "The Academy of Applied Osteopathy," and then in 1970 to it's present name, "The American Academy of Osteopathy" (AAO). It's functions are to arrange programs for education in OMT, to develop teachers of this concept, to publish papers on Osteopathic subjects, to discover persons with good manipulative skills, to promote research in Osteopathic Principles, and to serve the needs of it's members. A second organization, "The Osteopathic Cranial Association" was formed in 1946. It's purposes were the same as the American Academy of Osteopathy, but focused on the cranial aspect. It started as an independent organization, but then became a Component Society of the AAO. In 1960 the name was changed to it's present "Cranial Academy."

In the early years Osteopathy quickly spread to other areas in the world, but it was small and sporadic. In recent years this spread has become quite dramatic. Many foreign countries accept American trained D.O.'s, but some do not. Others such as England accept them, but limit their practice to just manipulation, which English trained D.O.'s are limited to. Many countries, with the help of American D.O.'s are training their own "Osteopaths," but they are limited to manipulation unless they have an M.D. degree. There are these limited Osteopathic Colleges in England (established many years ago), New Zealand, Canada, France, Belgium, Germany, and Japan. New Zealand has recently completed conversion to an Osteopathic Medical School. David A. Patriquin D.O., F.A.A.O., a 1956 graduate of the Philadelphia College of Osteopathic Medicine, who practiced in Montreal, Canada and was then on the faculty of the Ohio College of Osteopathic Medicine for many years, spent two years in New Zealand helping with the conversion.

In some foreign countries European M.D.'s have taken Osteopathic training and are allowed to practice "Osteopathy," some with licensure, some without. When they have obtained a Governmental Regulatory Agency, they may then become Associate Affiliate Members of the American Academy of Osteopathy, and attend our post-graduate courses. Other foreign "Osteopaths" start as Physical Therapists and take several thousand more hours of training in anatomy, physiology, chemistry, and manipulation. Their numbers are increasing rapidly, and some of them are quite proficient. They perhaps should be designated as "International Non-licensed Osteopaths."

This has caused some problems with the American Osteopathic Association, which in many ways has aligned itself with mainstream Medicine. The terms "Osteopathy" and "Osteopath" are historical terms directly linked with Dr. Still, the founder of Osteopathy. Some in the Osteopathic Profession would like to relegate the term "Osteopath" to historical perspective and only use the term "Osteopathic Physician." The two should be interchangeable. The American Academy of Osteopathy is vigorously defending the use of "Osteopath" and "Osteopathy."

11

Expanding the Concept

D r. Still had a definite mechanical aptitude and was able to build and repair mechanical devices. He invented a butter churn that greatly shortened the time required to churn butter out of cream. He invented the combine, but the idea was taken and patented by someone else. *(57)* He spoke of the human body as a machine, "Man, the most complex, intricate, and delicately constructed machine of all creation, is the one which the Osteopath must become familiar." *(ibid)* And he often spoke of God as the "Master mechanic."

When he developed his manual methods of treating diseases, he emphasized the inherent ability of the body to heal, and the importance of all parts working together in harmony. After opening the first school of Osteopathy in Kirksville, Missouri in 1892, Dr. Still in his teaching emphasized his philosophy and did not dwell on specific manipulative procedures, of which there are many. Osteopathic manipulative technics are applied to all of the tissues in the body wherever abnormalities are found. These tissues include the articulations or joints between bones, which include the spine, the arms, hands and fingers, the legs, feet and toes, and even the sutures or joints between the cranial bones. Much of the Medical Profession does not yet recognize that there is motion in the cranium, but it has only been in the last 50 years that they have recognized there is motion in the sacro-iliacs. We will discuss cranial motion in the next chapter.

These tissues also include the ligaments which support and limit the motion of joints, muscles which move and also support joints, tendons which attach muscles to bone, and fascias, the connective tissue which envelops all the tissues in the body and gives the body much of it's form. The fluids of the body are also treated. This includes the lymphatic fluid which is filtered from blood serum and bathes all of the tissues in the body, the blood contained in the arteries and veins, and the cerebro-spinal fluid which is in and around the brain and spinal cord. We also treat the brain through the cranial mechanism, the 12 pairs of special cranial nerves, the sympathetic and para-sympathetic nervous systems, and all the spinal nerves as they exit from the spine. The skin which covers everything also receives attention.

The abnormalities we look for are also numerous. These may be restricted motion in any of the bones mentioned above. Years ago we referred to such restrictions as "Osteopathic lesions," but they are now referred to as "somatic dysfunctions." We also look for increased or decreased tension in muscles, ligaments and fascia. We look for degenerative changes such as arthritis of joints, fibrositis of muscles and fascias, and dryness of the skin. We look for changes in blood and nerve supply as evidenced by congestion, inflammation, coldness, and impaired function of many kinds.

Because of the variety of tissues to be treated and the myriad of problems which may present themselves, there are a great number of manipulative procedures used. All are designed to improve function and help the body heal itself. All of the major manipulative procedures in use throughout the world today originated with the Osteopathic Profession, but many are being used by other health-care providers, with varying degrees of success.

The best known manipulative procedure is called direct action or high velocity low amplitude (HVLA). It is applied to restricted bony joints when indicated. It must be done with care or the patient can be injured. It should not be used in the presence of recent trauma, acute infections, advanced arthritic changes, osteoporosis, general debility, the very young, the very old, or patient apprehension. Joints may be restricted in their normal neutral position by thickening of ligaments or tightening of muscles, or they may be out of place in one or more of their ranges of motion - flexion (bending), extension (straightening), and sidebending and rotation. A careful examination must be done to determine exactly how that articulation varies from normal, in order to know how to treat it. Medicare and insurance companies don't have a clue about how important this evaluation is before initiating treatment. Then the soft tissues around the joint must be relaxed as much as possible so they are not strained in the correction, and the joint will move more easily. For best results, all of the components of the malformation must be reversed. When that repositioning is achieved, and when the slack has been taken up in the supportive tissues, a quick (high velocity) thrust back towards normal, with a short travel distance (low amplitude) is applied to restore normal motion and position. Persons who apply both a high velocity and a high amplitude (long travel distance) are very apt to injure their patient.

One of the best ways to relax and prepare the soft tissues, the skin, fascias and muscles is a technic called "soft tissue." The tissues are slowly and gently stretched away from the restricted area. When carefully and thoughtfully done, it is relaxing to the patient, and gives the operator a great deal of information about the patient, such as whether there has been an injury either recent or ancient, how adequate the patient's nutrition is, whether they are under undue stress, if they have an infection, whether or not they are getting exercise. This information is very helpful in understanding and addressing the patients problems.

Articulatory procedures may be applied to joints, which are

both mobilizing and corrective. These are applied by stabilizing the normal structure adjacent to a restricted one, and then moving the restriction either with direct contact to that part or moving the body part the restriction is a part of. These are gentle and have a wide application.

Then there are very gentle technics applied to fascias and ligaments to balance the tensions found in those structures. These are known as myo-fascial and ligamentous release. The approach may be direct or indirect depending on whether the problem is recent or chronic.

Body fluids may also be influenced in many ways. When an accumulation of lymph or tissue fluid is present, called edema, often occurring in the feet and ankles, the body part may be moved rhythmically to simulate muscular activity which normally keeps fluids circulating. This rhythmic pulsation helps the body get the accumulated fluid back into the circulatory system. An area with edema may also be gently stroked back towards the heart to reduce the swelling. A rhythmic pumping of the chest, called lymphatic pump will greatly reduce congestion in the lungs in respiratory diseases.

These are the main types of technic used in Dr. Still's day. Other methods have been added in more recent years, which will be discussed later in this chapter. There is still some debate about what kinds of procedures Dr. Still used, because his writings were mainly philosophy, and not specific technics, but there is ample evidence that he used a variety of different technics. It is quite clear that he used HVLA, high velocity low amplitude. He was known as the "lightning bone-setter." When D.D. Palmer spent two weeks with Dr. Still in 1893, and was treated by Dr. Still, then went back to Davenport, Iowa to announce his discovery of "Chiropractic." Palmer only used high velocity. Many of Dr. Still's early students published books and write specifically about HVLA. One such student was Edythe Ashmore, D.O. who became a professor of Osteopathic technic for Dr. Still, and published "Osteopathic Mechanics" *(70)* in 1915. She describes HVLA in her book, along with articulatory technics. Ernest E. Tucker, D.O., another professor at the American School of Osteopathy in his book, "Osteopathic Technic" *(71)* again specifically describes HVLA technics.

There were some more vigorous technics used where parts of the patients body were immobilized with straps, and adjacent areas were then manipulated. Early Osteopathic treatment tables, the McManus table manufactured in Kirksville, had several appendages for the attachment of straps. Joseph Swart, D.O., LL.B., an early graduate of The American School of Osteopathy, and later a professor at Kansas City, published a book "Osteopathic Strap Technic" *(72)* on this type of technic. Dr. D. L. Clark, a 1898 graduate of The American School of Osteopathy whom I mentioned in Chapter 9 was a master of strap technic. It was almost a lost art, but is being re-introduced.

Dr. Still also used articulatory technics, which were recorded in several books by his early students. It is also apparent that Dr. Still used some very gentle indirect technics directed at ligamentous and fascial structures. These are less definitive, employ almost imperceptible movements, and are not as easily understood. There are fewer references to these technics in early Osteopathic texts, but many of Dr. Still's pupils relied heavily on these gentle and very effective technics. One of the most outstanding was William Garner Sutherland, D.O. a 1900 graduate of A.S.O., the American School of Osteopathy. The next chapter is devoted to Dr. Sutherland and his very significant contribution to the expanding Osteopathic concept.

It is my feeling that Dr. Still concentrated on teaching his philosophy rather than on specific technics for two main reasons. First of all his approach was radically new and a total departure from the existing practice of medicine. His expressed desire was to "Improve the practice of medicine, surgery and obstetrics," *(57)* but he realized to be successful there would have to be a complete change in thinking. Secondly, I am sure he realized those that understood his new philosophy would develop other methods of application, and indeed this has been the case. Many D.O.'s have developed individual technics of their own, have somewhat modified existing methods, and have broadened the scope of existing methods, but there have been several who have produced entirely new methods.

In the 1940's a very specialized form of manipulation was developed by C. Haddon Soden, D.O. who graduated from A.S.O. in 1924, in the same class as my parents. Dr. Soden pioneered Manipulation Under Anesthesia. This is done in difficult cases, often chronic cases, and requires a very competent manipulator, and assistant to help move the patient, and a competent anesthesiologist because of the deep surgical anesthesia. The anesthesia completely obliterates the muscle protection of joints, so it is necessary for the operator to be completely familiar with the feel of the ligamentous structures. In keeping with the Osteopathic Philosophy, the whole musculo-skeletal system is mobilized.. Years ago I had Hospital Staff privileges to do this procedure and did dozens of cases. Some M.D. Orthopedic Surgeons do some manipulation under anesthesia, but usually single joints such as frozen shoulders. Lacking the "feel" of the tissues, they have often fractured the patients arm, and some Orthopedic Texts advise against doing such procedures.

In the early 50's Harold Hoover, D.O. and Charles Bowles, D.O. introduced Functional Technic. This involved using a "listening" or "feeling" hand over an affected area of the musculoskeletal system, waiting to "tune in" to what the tissues were doing, and then using a second hand to move an adjacent part back into harmony, or to guide the patient in a directed movement. This required supreme concentration on the part of the operator, and careful cooperation on the part of the patient. Because of it's complexity it did not gain very wide usage.

Another 1900 graduate, T.J. Ruddy, D.O., who practiced in

California for many years, and was the first Eye, Ear, Nose and Throat specialist, developed the "Resistive Duction" technics. This required repeated gentle muscular efforts on the part of the patient, against gentle resistance by the operator, and timed to be synchronous with the patient's heart beat. This was very effective for both improving restricted motion, and improving circulation, but did not gain wide acceptance.

Also in the 1950's a new and very effective technic called "Muscle Energy" was developed by Fred Mitchell, Sr., D.O. It has three different methods of application. In the first, a restricted joint is positioned as in direct action to reverse all it's abnormal components, it is moved up to the point of tension, and then the patient is directed to exert a gentle force in the opposite direction, with resistance from the operator so no motion is allowed. This muscular effort is held for 4 to 5 seconds, the patient is told to relax, the produced slack is taken up, and the procedure is repeated till a satisfactory release is obtained. Dr. Mitchell called this portion "Iso-metric." It can also be used for muscle conditioning. A second application is primarily to strengthen muscles. In this procedure the patient exerts a gentle force and the operator exerts a lesser resistance, so motion is introduced. This is also sustained for 4 to 5 seconds, and then repeated. Dr. Mitchell called this "Iso-tonic." The third application is directed at a muscle or muscle group that is tense and fibrotic. The patient again exerts a muscle action against the operator, but the operator exerts a greater force so motion is introduced in the opposite direction providing a very effective stretching. Dr. Mitchell was still developing the concept when he taught at a post-graduate meeting at the offices I shared with my father. Dr. Mitchell had not come up with a name for this third application, and I suggested "Iso-lytic" which he liked and adopted. Muscle Energy is a very effective procedure, has a common principle that can be applied anywhere in the body, and is widely used. In recent times it has been modified in some ways by Fred Mitchell, Jr. D.O. who is on the faculty of the Michigan State College of Osteopathic Medicine. In the 1960's Larry Jones . D.O., developed "Counter-Strain." This was originally developed to reverse acute strains by placing the patient in the position they were in when the strain occurred, holding them there for 90 seconds to let the muscle relax, and then slowly and gently returning them to a neutral position with operator effort only. It's scope has been broadened to treat other dysfunctions, and is widely used by many health care providers.

Osteopathic Physicians also direct various types of manipulation to internal organs that are accessible. For instance congested livers can be carefully pumped through the rib cage to improve the metabolism of food, increase detoxification, and improve other liver functions. In the 1930's Yale Castlio, D.O. and Louise Ferris-Smith demonstrated that pumping the spleen will increase circulating white blood cells and anti-bodies. *(73)* This is a very helpful procedure in both infectious processes and allergic problems. All of the abdominal and pelvic organs can be influenced by gentle application through the abdominal wall termed "Ventral Technic." A mal-positioned uterus can be repositioned by gentle intra-pelvic technic.

All organs of the body, those accessible externally and those not accessible, can be influenced through their blood and nerve supply, which when impaired will cause functional changes in that organ. This was the basis of the research done by Dr. Louisa Burns in the early 1900's, to show the pathologic effects of impaired blood and nerve supply on internal organs, and to provide some proof of the Osteopathic concept. Every organ in the body has a specific segmental innervation from the spinal cord, which is consistent in every individual. This is documented in every anatomy book. What was not documented was that when an organ becomes diseased, it sets up a reaction in the spinal cord at the level of it's innervation, which then affects the voluntary nerves at that same level. These reflex connections were mapped out by

Francis Pottenger M.D., FCAP in his classic text, "Symptoms of Visceral Disease." *(74)* He was ridiculed by his own Medical Profession, and his membership was rescinded. Years later when greater knowledge of the nervous system proved him right, he was taken back with honors. We use these spinal reflexes in Osteopathic Medicine both diagnostically and therapeutically. A restricted area of the spine will affect the autonomic nerve supply to whatever organ is innervated by that segment. This is termed a "somato-visceral" reflex, the somato referring to the somatic or supporting structures of the body, and the visceral referring to the visceral organ. On the other hand, if an internal organ is damaged by disease or trauma, a reflex is also set up to the spinal cord, which is termed a viscero-somatic reflex. This will be evidenced by tension in the deep spinal muscles at that segment and can be palpated with a trained sense of touch. This gives valuable information about what is going on in the body. In treating a patient, if they have not mentioned any symptoms, but you find tension in the area of nerve supply to the stomach for instance, and ask, "have you had any stomach problems?" the patient will often answer, "yes, how did you know?" Treating the irritated spinal segment will usually relieve the symptoms.

Another set of entirely different reflexes were discovered around the turn of the century by Frank Chapman, D.O. They are described as "neuro-lymphatic" reflexes found in superficial lymphoid tissue with nerve endings related to all viscera and endocrine glands. They are still not completely understood, but for every "itis" there is a specific Chapman's reflex whether it be sinusitis, colitis, thyroiditis or whatever. They are very helpful diagnostically when they are located because Dr. Chapman mapped over 200 such reflexes. And once located they can be treated to improve the condition they are related to.

Dr. Mitchell, the developer of Muscle Energy was introduced to Osteopathy because of Chapman's Reflexes. He was a business man in Chattanooga, Tennessee. Their home was damaged by a fire, and their two year old son was badly burned. The son's condition worsened, and when his kidneys stopped functioning, the M.D.s in attendance said it would only be a matter of hours before the boy died. The Mitchells had heard of a Dr. Owens, who had been working with Dr. Chapman, and asked if they could call him in consultation. The M.D.s replied that it wouldn't really matter, the boy was going to die anyway. After arriving, Dr. Owens assessed the situation and then treated the Chapman's Reflexes for the kidneys, the adrenal glands, and the liver. In about 30 minutes the boys kidneys resumed functioning, and later Dr. Mitchell recalled it was the most foul smelling stuff he had ever smelled. The boy regained his health, which so inspired Mr. Mitchell that he sold his business and studied Osteopathy, becoming one of our outstanding members. The son, Fred Mitchell Jr, D.O., F.A.A.O. is one of our professions most respected members and is on the Faculty of the Michigan State College of Osteopathic Medicine.

Shortly after hearing Dr. Mitchell lecture about Chapman's Reflexes and relate his son's story years ago, my father-in law became seriously ill due to a bowel obstruction. This was back in the 1950's when diagnostic measures were much more limited. The surgeon I had called in consultation was an excellent diagnostician. With my father-in laws age, and because he drank and smoked, we figured the obstruction was probably a malignancy. During surgery however we found something had perforated the bowel wall, perhaps a fish bone, and a large abscess had formed which had blocked his bowel. We drained the abscess, removed the adhesions that had formed, and sewed him up. He seemed to be doing all right, but two days later his wound burst open (eviscerated) and he had a massive peritonitis, an infection of the lining of the abdomen. The surgeon gave him no chance at all to survive these complications. I immediately called Dr. Mitchell and asked him what reflexes to work on, and he replied "liver, adrenals, kidneys, and bowel." For the next week I went to the hospital morning , noon and night to work on Chapman's Reflexes, and my father-in law regained his health. The Osteopathic Profession has many stories like this in it's rich tradition.

12

The Cranio–Sacral Concept of William Garner Sutherland, D.O.

T he greatest contribution to the expanding Osteopathic Concept, and one of the greatest blessings to health care deserves a chapter of it's own. This is the Dr. Sutherland's Cranio-Sacral Concept. Some still think of it as something "extra," or something "different," but it is the most important part of the Osteopathic Philosophy even though it came along years after Dr. Still's original work. Dr. Still set the ground work when he made such statements as "the cerebro-spinal fluid is the highest known element in the human body," *(57)* and "unless the brain furnishes this fluid in abundance, a disabled condition of the body will remain." *(ibid)* One old-time Osteopath who has learned the cranio-sacral concept remarked, "until cranial came along we were practicing decerebrate Osteopathy." It's importance lies in the fact that the cranio-sacral mechanism affects all of the functions of the brain and spinal cord, it affects the master gland of the endocrine system, the pituitary gland, and it affects the flow of the cerebro-spinal fluid with the distribution of the neuro-transmitters produced by the brain.

Will Sutherland grew up in farm country in Troy, Minnesota. His father was a blacksmith, but grew much of his own food. One of Will's chores was to dig potatoes with his older brother. One year after digging what they thought was an adequate harvest, their father told them, "go dig again, boys." So they dug some more and found more potatoes, but after surveying the potato patch, their father said, "go dig again, boys." Again they harvested more potatoes. This taught Will a lesson which stayed with him throughout life, that "it pays to dig on." *(75)* The family later moved to Blunt, South Dakota and they were now a family of six. The boys were obliged to go to work to help support the family. Will became a "printer's devil" or odd-job boy for the local newspaper, the Blunt Advocate. Will was conscientious, hard working, had good mechanical sense, and a good sense of humor. After working in the newspaper business for a number of years, Will realized that he needed more education and enrolled at Upper Iowa University, but returned to the newspaper business before he had graduated.

Will first learned about Osteopathy while working for the Austin Daily Herald in Minnesota. He had a close friend whose family were well acquainted with Dr. and Mrs. Still. His interest was heightened when his older brother was restored to health by Osteopathy. He then had the opportunity to visit Kirksville, and as was natural for a newspaper reporter, talked to students, patients and doctors. He was so impressed by what he heard that he decided to make it his life's work, a choice for which he was always grateful. He enrolled in 1898 in a class of 162 which was quite a change from the class of 18 just six years earlier. One day in school he was looking at a disarticulated skull. This is a skull in which the 22 bones have been taken apart, but held in relative position by little braces so their relationships can be studied. All Osteopathic and Medical Schools have such a specimen. Dr.

Sutherland later recalled, "As I stood looking and thinking in the channel of Dr. Still's philosophy, my attention was called to the beveled articular surface of the sphenoid bone. Suddenly there came a thought - I call it a guiding thought - beveled like the gills of a fish, indicating articular mobility for a respiratory mechanism." *(75)* Then he started asking himself how crazy that line of thinking was. He could find no substantiation for his thought, because most anatomy books stated that the bones fused in adult life, and they still do so state. But here in front of Will Sutherland was a specimen, with hundreds or even more just like it in Medical Schools around the World, graphically demonstrating that the bones do not fuse, and can be taken apart! In his two years in Osteopathic School, all that was required at that time, similar to Medical Schools, it was apparent to Will that he must keep digging in his Osteopathic studies. He also responded more than others to Dr. Still's insistence on knowing anatomy. Will described Dr. Still as "a profound and honest thinker, philosopher and humanitarian; as a man who walked closely with God." *(75)*

Will tried to get the idea of cranial motion out of his mind, thinking it was senseless, but it kept recurring. His attention was diverted upon his graduation in 1900 with the necessity of getting a practice started, which he did in a room of his parents home. After a few months he was successful enough to rent an office and proudly hung his sign, "Dr. William G. Sutherland, Osteopath." *(ibid)* In his training from Dr. Still he had picked up the importance of feeling the tissues being worked on. Dr. Sutherland made that a part of his practice more than any other Osteopathic graduate, and developed his famous "thinking, seeing, feeling fingers." *(ibid)* In later years he also added "knowing." The thought of cranial motion kept hounding him, and he worked diligently at developing his sense of touch.

His newspaper days made it natural for him to start writing. One of his first articles was, "Let's Be Up and Touching," *(ibid)* saying, "Osteopathic technic is governed by and through the intelligent application of the intelligent sense of touch." *(ibid)* Finally in the 1920's he could no longer ignore the gnawing question in his mind, was there motion in the skull? The usual method of disarticulating a skull was to put dried beans in the skull and then soak it in water and have the force of the expanding beans force the bones apart, which again demonstrates that the boned do not fuse. This was too crude for Dr. Sutherland, so he took a pen knife and carefully pried the bones apart, closely studying each articulation. With the same mechanical sense that Dr. Still had, Dr. Sutherland related the cranial sutures to gears, ball and socket joints, pulleys, fulcrums, and other mechanical devices, and was sure that such devices were designed for rocking, gliding, rotations, and other types of motion. But this was only theory and needed to be proven. Then he reasoned that the stoutest oak tree will bend in the wind, but when dead and dried is very rigid. About this time Dr. Sutherland met a very wonderful woman, Adah Strand. He had been previously married, but was divorced. Adah proved to be a great helper and supporter. They were married on May 22nd, 1924, and spent their honeymoon in Kirksville where they were celebrating the "A. T. Still Jubilee, 1874 - 1924." As a part of the celebration the annual convention of the American Osteopathic Association was held in Kirksville. And there was an interesting coincidence. Both of my parents were graduating from Kirksville (The American School of Osteopathy) at that same time. Little did they know that years later they would become very close to the Sutherlands.

Further reasoning suggested to Dr. Sutherland that since the base of the skull is formed in cartilage which later ossifies, and that the vault (top of the skull) is formed in membrane which also later ossifies, this must indicate an adaptive arrangement for motion. He felt that the membranes which line the inside of the skull, the meninges, with several projections which separate and support portions of the brain, are the controlling mechanism of the bones. He named this controlling mechanism "The Reciprocal Tension Membrane." *(ibid)* He realized that he had to prove his theory, but being as dedicated as he was, felt strongly that he needed to feel it himself. He constantly had cranial bones around the house so he could become completely familiar with every one of them. Then he started experimenting with his own head. Talk about "digging on!" Being quite mechanically inclined, just as Dr. Still was, he built devices out of all sorts of things such as wooden bowls, football helmets, baseball gloves, rubber bands, leather straps - all designed to jam certain sutures in his own head so he could see and feel what symptoms it caused. He enlisted the help of Mrs. Sutherland, which caused her great alarm at times, but he knew his anatomy well enough he could undo the damage with her help. His delicate sense of touch told him that there was indeed motion in the cranial mechanism, and since it was already known that there was motion in the brain, he realized that the skull has to move to accommodate the motion of the brain and fluctuation of cerebro-spinal fluid. Then he found an anatomy book that stated that all of the physiologic centers of the brain, including that for respiration, are in the floor of the 4th ventricle, one of the openings in the brain. He then concluded that the mechanism he was studying was actually a primary respiratory mechanism, and the respiration of the lungs was secondary. This has proven to be true. Dr. Sutherland continued his research in every way possible, studying the minute relationships of the bones, still experimenting with his own head and sacrum (tailbone), and found that the sacrum had respiratory motion and was closely tied to the cranium. He called this the cranio-sacral mechanism.

Dr. Sutherland also spent time observing peoples heads. It was said that he made many strangers uncomfortable in public by staring at their heads. Then he started correlating his cranial findings in patients with remarks they made about head injuries and bumps they had suffered. Finally he carefully started treating patients with his new methods, and got good results. Migraine headaches were a common problem, and also sinus infections and eye problems. Following Dr. Still's teachings, he studied the tissues of all the body, and applied his gentle approach to all parts of the body, wherever he found problems. At this point he felt it was time to "spread the word." He wrote a series of articles in an Osteopathic Publication titled, "Skull Notions by Blunt Bone Bill," undoubtedly harking back to his upbringing in Blunt, South Dakota. He was asked to lecture at the 1932 A.O.A. Convention in Chicago. Only seven attended, but it did create some interest. To this point his efforts had been directed to adults, but patients were asking about their children with problems. Dr. Sutherland realized that many problems arise from birth trauma, when the bones are soft and pliable which allows for some molding to make the birth process easier. The 22 bones which make up the adult skull, develop in two, three, even four parts in the infant, and later fuse into one bone. This prompted Dr. Sutherland to apply to the results of birth trauma Alexander Pope's famous lines "'Tis education forms the common mind; just as the twig is bent, the tree's inclined." *(74)* Realizing what a great need there was for these "bent twigs," but also realizing his limited experience, Dr. Sutherland started spending 2 days a week in Minneapolis-St. Paul at children's clinic devoted to eye and speech problems. He kept this up for 5 years, at great personal sacrifice, but with great rewards in knowledge and benefit to handicapped children.

In 1939 he published a booklet titled "The Cranial Bowl" which did not sell well, but did lead to a series of lectures. One was at the 1940 A.O.A. Convention in Chicago, which caught the attention of two prominent members of the Academy of Applied Osteopathy, Dr. Perrin Wilson who had been my father's family doctor in Boston and was the reason my father elected to study Osteopathy. The other was Dr. Tom Northup who was instrumental in forming the Academy of Applied Osteopathy, now the American Academy of Osteopathy. Several doctors had been studying with Dr. Sutherland, most noteworthy of which were Drs. Howard and Rebecca Lippincott. They helped Dr. Sutherland publish a workbook.

In 1944 a big breakthrough occurred when Dr. Sutherland was asked to put on a class at the Des Moines Still Osteopathic College. This was facilitated by Dr. Paul Kimberly who was teaching anatomy at the college at that time. This was the first of many classes to follow. With many new doctors learning the concept, it became important to have an organization to serve their needs. Drs. Wilson and Northup were instrumental in forming the Osteopathic Cranial Association in 1947.

In 1946 an interesting twist of fate occurred. My father, Harold Magoun Sr., D.O., F.A.A.O. had fallen ice skating as a child, had struck the back of his head, and suffered severe migraine headaches for many years. He had heard of some nuts in the profession who were talking about motion in the cranium, when everyone knew it was a solid bony case. He signed up for one of the classes to expose the charlatans. By this time Dr. Sutherland had done such a detailed study of the cranium, he could do a visual diagnosis in many cases. The minute my father walked into the room, Dr. Sutherland asked him how long he had suffered from migraine headaches. This of course caught my father's attention and changed his line of thinking. During the rest of that week, under Dr. Sutherland's direction, Drs. Tom Schooley, Ken Little, and Reginald Platt, who had been studying with Dr. Sutherland, worked on my father's head. They used multiple-hand technic, got my father's head freed up, and he never had another migraine. In a situation where several cranially trained doctors are available, two or three can work on the head, one on the sacrum, even someone on the lower extremities can affect the cranio-sacral mechanism. This is all done under careful guidance by the most experienced member of the group and accomplishes much more than one individual can do by himself. My father then became a devoted disciple of Dr. Sutherlands, worked with him for a number of years, and compiled Dr. Sutherland's teachings into the first text on cranial manipulation, "Osteopathy in the Cranial Field," (77) first published in 1951, with two subsequent editions in 1966 and 1976. My father spent thousands of hours in writing the book with suggestions from early notables such as Drs. Ann Wales, Rollin Becker, and the Lippincotts. He stated in the book, "This is a labor of love - an attempt to pay back an obligation for relief from pain, with no remuneration asked or received." *(ibid)* The book was donated to the Cranial Academy. As his legal heir, I now hold the copyright. As Osteopathy spreads throughout the world, "Osteopathy in the Cranial Field" has now been translated into French, German, Italian, and Japanese.

Desiring to preserve the purity of Dr. Sutherland's teachings, the Sutherland Cranial Teaching Foundation was incorporated in Denver on September 25, 1953, with Dr. William G. Sutherland President, Dr. Harold Magoun Sr. Executive Vice President, Mrs. Adah Sutherland Vice President, and Dr. Chester Handy Secretary-Treasurer. The organization has a Board of Trustees, conducts post-graduate teaching seminars, but has no membership organization. Dr. Sutherland passed away on September 23, 1954 in Pacific Grove, California. He left a tremendous living legacy.

Dr. Sutherland's theory and subsequent findings proved several things about the skull, brain, spinal cord and sacrum:

1. The brain slightly coils and uncoils 10 to 12 times a minute normally.

2. There is pliability to living cranial bones, there is motion in the cranial sutures, and these sutures are definitely joints. Subsequent research, particularly in the United States and in Russia, has shown that the dura mater, the tough membrane that lines the inside of the skull and has several reflexions which separate and support portions of the brain, is continuous through the sutures with the periosteum, the connective tissue which lines

the outside of all bones. These joint surfaces or sutures also have blood and nerve supply.

3. The dura mater, especially it's reflexions, has inherent tensions in it which controls the motion in the cranial bones.

4. The dura mater, which covers the brain and the spinal cord, is attached to the base of the skull, surrounds the spinal cord throughout it's whole length, and then is attached to the sacrum (tail bone). The dura, being inelastic, exerts tension on both the base of the skull and the sacrum, so changes in motion on one end will affect the other. This is the basis of the cranio-sacral mechanism. Dr. Sutherland made the analogy of the old-fashioned clothes line, with two "T" poles set in the ground, and wires running between the two arms. Pulling on one arm of the post will then pull on the arm at the other end.

5. The sacrum also moves between the hip bones as part of the Primary Respiratory Mechanism. This is independent of the gross movement which is part of the walking cycle.

6. The cerebro-spinal fluid fluctuates like the tides of the ocean, but also circulates and flows along all of the cranial and spinal nerves.

This is a tremendous departure from traditional medical and dental thinking, which is slow to change. Some M.D.'s who do manipulation called "manual medicine" have taken Osteopathic Cranial courses and make cranio-sacral manipulation part of their practices. Andrew Weil, M.D., author of "Spontaneous Healing," *(7)* relates in his book how he discovered Robert Fulford, D.O., one of Dr. Sutherlands most outstanding pupils, observed the results of cranio-sacral treatment, and experienced it himself. Dr. Weil now recommends cranio-sacral treatment in his newsletter, "Self Healing." (78) Dr. Weil is to be greatly admired for being open-minded and being a leader in holistic medicine. Dr. Fulford was loved by his patients, and greatly admired by his profession. Many years ago at a Cranial conference in Whittier, California, which I attended, Dr. Fulford was on the program. There had been lectures in the morning, and just before lunch was a question and answer period. One of the registrants directed a question to Dr. Fulford about what to do for a newborn infant that wouldn't nurse. Dr. Fulford responded that on his way to the airport he had been asked to stop by the hospital to treat just such an infant. He described what he had done, and stated that in 15 minutes the baby was nursing. There was an awed silence, and then the registrant said, "but what about us mortals?" Such was the respect for Dr. Fulford.

Many dentists have also taken our Osteopathic post-graduate courses in cranio-sacral manipulation and find it to be very essential in the proper treatment of tempero-mandibular-joint disease, mal-occlusion, facial pain, and other problems they deal with. Treating the sacrum presents some problems for a dentist. Some of them will, but others prefer to refer the patient to a competent Osteopath. However, a number of years ago the Appellate Court ruled in Colorado that a Dentist trained in cranio-sacral treatment can properly treat the sacrum under the provisions of the Colorado Dental Practice Act. I was asked to testify in that court case, and it was a landmark decision. We have many M.D. and Dentist members in the Cranial Academy.

For many years the Upledger Institute in Florida has been training physical therapists to do "cranio-sacral therapy," and indeed it is just therapy. Some of these physical therapists have then been teaching anyone who will pay the registration fee for a class. This is a terrible mistake. Many people can be taught to do the mechanics of cranial manipulation, and some of them develop a feel for the tissues, but lacking the background Osteopathic, Medical or Dental education, they do not understand the many indicational and contra-indications for doing the delicate work it entails, and they have hurt many people. This is a shame, and should not be.

In the next chapter we will discuss many of the conditions which benefit from cranio-sacral treatment.

13

Osteopathic Contributions to Health Care

D r. Still was a true family practitioner. He successfully treated diseases of all kinds - pneumonia, chicken pox, small pox, cholera, typhoid, measles, mumps, whooping cough, bloody flux (which we now would call colitis), eye problems, many unidentified neurological diseases, and many kinds of sprains and soft tissue diseases. His success was what made Osteopathy grow so rapidly. He was successful for several reasons. Even though life-expectancy was not as long as it is now, his patients were not affected by air pollution, radiation, the refined foods, and the thousands of hazardous chemicals we are exposed to which constantly assault our immune system and our neuro-musculo-skeletal systems. In Dr. Still's day, the worst thing was the very poisonous drugs being prescribed by the doctors! Dr. Still understood how the body functioned, had learned every bone, artery and nerve, knew where to look for trouble, and had learned how to correct the problems he found, so his patients responded to his new method of treatment. He did not preach health-care without drugs or surgery, but wanted to minimize their use because he had found methods that were more effective in many instances. His desire was "to improve the practice of medicine, surgery and obstetrics." *(57)*

The Osteopathic Profession is an interesting one. At one time all Osteopathic Physicians used OMT (Osteopathic Manipulative Treatment) in their practices, including the specialists. Now days some don't, and statistics vary as to the exact percentages. There is probably no profession where there is a greater variety in levels of skill. Some have been extremely skilled, several of whom I have mentioned such as Dr. Perrin Wilson, Dr. Fred Mitchel Sr., Dr. Harrison Freyette, Dr. William Sutherland, Dr. Rollin Becker, Drs. Howard and Rebecca Lippincott, Dr. Harold Magoun Sr., and Dr. Robert Fulford. I will only mention some who have already passed on. Others who use some manipulation are rather crude at it, either lacking the mechanical aptitude necessary, or just not having applied themselves, but as one old-time Osteopath said many years ago, "Osteopathy is so good, any damn fool can make a living at it." We also have skilled specialists in all fields of medicine and surgery, some of whom do use some manipulation. We have Certifying Boards in all of those specialties. Then we have a Certifying Board which the M.D.'s do not have, in Manipulation. For several years it was the "American Osteopathic Board of Special Proficiency in Osteopathic Manipulative Medicine," but has been changed by the American Osteopathic Association to the "American Osteopathic Board of Neuro-Musculo-Skeletal Medicine." Having qualified in that, with additional training and experience, and passing some demanding examinations, one can become a Fellow of the American Academy of Osteopathy." (F.A.A.O.)

The largest group in our profession are the Family Practitioners, who also have a Certifying Board. Many of them do some OMT, but some with complete practice rights just practice Medicine. They are in no sense family practitioners as Dr. Still was.

The group who most closely follow and maintain Dr. Still's

teachings are the members of The American Academy of Osteopathy (A.A.O.), and it's component society, The Cranial Academy (C.A.). Both organizations are very active in promoting
Osteopathy and serving the needs of their members. Both have
outstanding Executive Directors, Stephen J. Noone of the A.A.O.,
and Mrs. Pat Crampton of the Cranial Academy. Members of
these two Academies are devoted to Osteopathy. Some do family
practice using OMT and prescribing some drugs, others just do
OMT, and Cranio-Sacral treatment. All of this leads to an identity crisis. Just what is an Osteopathic Physician, or an Osteopath? One of my purposes in writing this book is to clarify that
question. A D.O. is a Doctor of Osteopathy. We are fully licensed
to practice Medicine Surgery and Obstetrics in all 50 States, but
we have additional training in Osteopathic Principles and Practice so we more fully understand how the body works, and how
all it's systems are closely related. With our training in palpation
we are able to " tune in" to the body and get valuable information about what is wrong. Then we have a variety of Osteopathic
procedures which help the body heal itself. I have already mentioned that the Medical Profession is investigating adding manipulation, or "Manual Medicine" as they call it to the Medical
School curricula, realizing that they have a deficiency. Those
D.O.'s who just practice medicine have missed the boat and are
denying their patients the most beneficial and cost-effective treatment in the majority of medical problems. By going to a medical
practice they may think they are "going modern," but in reality
they are old-fashioned, and have gone back to what Dr. Still escaped from, and became very successful with. Those of us who
do OMT are very proud to be known as Osteopaths, while those
who practice Medicine want to be known only as Osteopathic
Physicians. The use of Osteopathic Principles and Practice has
made Osteopathy grow and spread world-wide, not the practice
of medicine.

What can be treated with OMT of one kind or another? Remember that we have a great variety of procedures from very gentle indirect technics to very specific and potent direct technics. I can think of only one contra-indication for OMT of some kind. That is Tetanus, where even slight stimulation can set off violent muscle spasms. Tetanus is virtually unheard of because of the use of vaccination which supplements the body's immune system, and the use of tetanus anti-toxin in emergencies. Even in cancer, Dr. William Kelley who refined the Gerson (a German M.D.) cancer nutritional program, wants his patients carefully manipulated because he realizes that it enhances the body's immune system.

Lets discuss some of the health problems which benefit from OMT. And remember that good nutrition as outlined in Section I, will help the body overcome disease and injury, and improve response to OMT. I will mention a number of different health problems, and give a few examples from each group which OMT helps to correct. This will be far from a complete list, but should give you the idea.

Respiratory Disease

One of the most dramatic stories of the efficacy of OMT comes from the flu epidemic of World War I. This epidemic was spread from pigs to the Spanish Army, and is known as the swine flu. It quickly spread to other armies, then to the civilian population, and continued for two years. It caused between 21 and 25 million casualties, which at that time was 1% of the world's population, and was the worst epidemic on record. In the United States there were over 540,000 casualties. In the Military the mortality rate was 36%. In Medical Hospitals the mortality rate ranged between 30 and 40%, but was 68% in New York City, probably because of more crowded conditions. The American School of Osteopathy wrote to all their alumni and asked them to report on their treatment of flu cases. They received a response from 2,445 D.O.'s who had treated 110,122 cases with a mortality rate of 0.25 %. *(61)* Massachusetts Osteopathic Hospital, a 400 bed hospital also reported a 0.25 % mortality rate. Why the tremendous difference? The medical treatment was cough syrup and aspirin. The cough syrup loosened the cough, but the aspirin given to treat the fever as a symptom, impaired the body's normal response to an infection - elevation of temperature. The results were disastrous. The Osteopathic treatment was cough syrup and Osteopathic manipulation, which included "rib-raising" to improve breathing and circulation in the chest, "lymphatic pump" to reduce congestion in the chest, and other procedures to make the patient more comfortable and enhance the immune system. Several years ago a prominent M.D. here in Denver retired after many years in practice. In his memoirs he recounted coming to Denver during the flu epidemic, and was told to give cough syrup and aspirin. Unfortunately that same philosophy still exists today, with one change. Many doctors today treat flu with cough syrup, aspirin or tylenol, and an anti-biotic. It is well known that viruses are not affected by anti-biotics, but doctors go on treating symptoms. The anti-biotic in some cases may prevent a secondary bacterial infection, but this is poor medicine. By far the best treatment is OMT and vitamin C.

Pneumonia. Pulmonary congestion is usually more localized in pneumonia, but is apt to be worse than in flu. This also responds well to OMT.

The Common Cold. There is an old saying that it takes a doctor 7 days to cure a cold, but nature can do it in a week. This time can be shortened by OMT, especially when it includes cranial treatment to improve venous and lymphatic drainage from the head. Vitamins A and C are also very helpful. I also recommend that my patients avoid dairy products because of their mucous producing tendency. This is true for all respiratory infections.

Asthma responds very well to OMT.

Sinusitis. This is becoming more of a problem, both because of the evolution of more virulent bacteria, and the ineffectiveness of many anti-biotics from over-usage. It is more of a problem in dry climates such as we have in Colorado, because the mucous membranes dry out and lose much of their protective mechanism. A good humidifier is a must. Even though they are more trouble to clean, I prefer the steam vaporizers because they leave the minerals and any contaminates in the container. In 1991 Dr. Robert Ivker here in Denver published a good book, "Sinus Survival." *(79)* He thoroughly discusses what the sinuses are, their function, the symptoms of sinusitis, and things a person should do in changing their life-style to overcome sinus problems. I found the book very disappointing in one important aspect. Dr. Ivker is an Osteopathic Physician, but doesn't mention this till near the end of his book. The Forward and all testimonials are by M.D.'s. He barely mentions Osteopathy, and when he does it is "Osteopathic Manipulative Therapy," and "Cranio-Sacral Therapy." Osteopathic Physicians give "treatment" not therapy. This quite clearly demonstrates that he is Allopathically oriented, and is one who missed the boat as discussed earlier in this chapter. He has missed a golden opportunity to experience the beneficial effects of OMT, and spread the word to many others. Chapman's Reflexes for a well-trained Osteopath are very specific in diagnosing sinusitis without requiring X-rays, and are helpful in treatment. Cranio-Sacral treatment is very effective in improving drainage from the sinuses to relieve congestion and pain, and to improve circulation to the areas so the immune system can overcome the infection. Nutritional support is essential, with vitamin A to build up the mucous membranes, vitamin C to support the immune system, lots of water to help liquefy the mucous, and again avoiding dairy products.

Gastro–intestinal Problems

Stomach and bowel problems are very common. Some of the reasons are, so many people put things in their stomach that just shouldn't be there. We are exposed to so much stress and there are many connections from the emotional centers of the brain to the stomach which can disturb it's function. Then many people don't keep regular bowel habits for elimination. Constipation is one of the most common problems. Improper diet and lack of adequate fluid intake can contribute significantly to poor elimination. The involuntary nerve control of the bowel is a very important factor. The Sympathetic portion of the autonomic nervous system arises from a chain of nerves on either side of the thoracic spine (where the rib cage attaches). Stimulation of the lower portion of the sympathetic chain will tighten the sphincters which close the bowel, and inhibit the peristaltic muscle action which moves the bowel contents through the colon. OMT to the lower thoracic area and gentle ventral technic to the abdominal wall will normalize bowel function. For my patients with constipation I give them a hand-out, as follows:

H - develop the habit of emptying the bowel every morning.

A - activity in the form of good exercise will aid bowel function.

B - bulk in the diet is essential to give the bowel something to work on.

I - intake of adequate water is essential to keep the feces soft for easier elimination.

T - treatment (Osteopathic) will greatly aid bowel function.

On the other side of the coin, over-activity of the pelvic outflow of the Para-Sympathetic portion of the autonomic nervous system which controls the muscular peristaltic action will result in diarrhea. OMT to the pelvis is therefore indicated, and is very helpful.

Irritable Bowel Syndrome is very common. We frequently find dietary indiscretions, nutritional deficiencies, especially vitamin A which is important for the mucous membrane lining the bowel, and always problems in the lower thoracic spine affecting the sympathetic nerves. Chapman's reflexes are always present, and are small tender "shotty" areas down the side or front of the thigh in the superficial tissues. To an Osteopath these are diagnostic and can be treated to relieve the problem.

Flatulence, or gaseous distension of the stomach and bowel is distressing. Diet is usually a factor, and often a deficiency of natural digestive enzymes is part of the problem. Osteopathic treatment to normalize blood and nerve supply, some dietary changes, and supplemental digestive enzymes will usually solve the problem.

Cardiology

Everyone is concerned about their heart, as well they should be. Arrythmia or irregular heart beat is one of the most common problems. This is often due to interference of the autonomic nerve supply to the heart. I have always found problems in the upper thoracic area, especially at the third thoracic vertebra and associated ribs. OMT will nearly always correct the problem, but if it persists, a cardiologist should be consulted. Tachycardia, or rapid heart beat is another common problem, and usually responds to OMT, but again if it persists, a cardiologist should be consulted. Angina, or chest pain due to impaired circulation to the heart can usually be relieved by OMT. In more severe cases, OMT will usually lessen the need for medication, There are many instances where restriction of the upper ribs will cause chest pain which is mistaken for angina. The EKG will be negative, which is confusing, but OMT is the answer.

In more serious cases such as congestive heart failure and

coronary infarction, gentle OMT, even in the intensive care unit will improve the patients condition, and make medication and other supportive measures more effective.

Endocrinology

Endocrine glands are ductless glands, or glands of internal secretion where their hormone secretions are distributed by tissue fluids. The major ones are the pituitary, thyroid, parathyroid, adrenals, ovaries, and testes. Alterations of blood and nerve supply are responsible for many endocrine problems, and can be helped by appropriate OMT. Cranial treatment is especially important, because the pituitary gland, "the master gland," is suspended in the middle of the cranial mechanism, and influences all other endocrine glands.

Surgery

This is a very broad and inclusive area of health care. In many instances, OMT will improve function enough to eliminate the need for surgical intervention in many different conditions. This could include gallbladder disease, stomach ulcers, thoracic outlet syndrome (removal of the first rib), bowel resection, herniated discs, etc. Of course surgeons don't like to hear this.

When surgery is necessary, careful OMT in the hospital setting will keep the patient more comfortable, help prevent complications such as paralytic ileus (post-surgical paralysis of the small bowel), post-operative pneumonia, blood clots, venous and lymphatic stasis, and will hasten the convalescence. In the early 1970's, Edward Stiles, D.O., F.A.A.O. conducted some studies of OMT in the hospital setting at the Waterville Osteopathic Hospital in Waterville, Maine. *(80)* He demonstrated the following decrease in hospital stay for patients who received OMT as compared to similar patients who did not receive OMT. Cholecystectomies (removal of gallbladder) 7%, appendectomies 40%, uncomplicated hysterectomies 12%, and complicated hysterectomies 22%. This represents a great benefit to the patient, and a significant reduction in the cost of the hospital stay. I interned at Rocky Mountain Osteopathic Hospital here in Denver in 1950-51. It was a small hospital, and there were only two interns for the first 6 months. The other intern was Walter Mill, D.O., F.A.A.O., F.A.C.O.S. who is now retired from the faculty of the Michigan State University College of Osteopathic Medicine. Dr. Mill and I did rib-raising and soft tissue on every surgical patient every day, and we had no cases of post-operative pneumonia. The last figures I saw showed a national average of 4% mortality from post-surgical pneumonia.

Psychiatry

OMT has a great deal to offer in nervous and mental diseases. Arthur G. Hildreth D.O., a graduate of the first class of the American School of Osteopathy in 1894, and a close friend of Dr. Still's, found a relationship of restriction at the 4th thoracic (between the shoulder blades) and the first cervical (the topmost vertebra in the neck) with depression. I have found this to be very consistent. Dr. Hildreth became interested in nervous and mental diseases, and in 1914 established the Still-Hildreth Osteopathic Sanatorium in Macon, Missouri for treatment of mental illness. This operated very successfully for many years. They employed standard psychiatric care with OMT, with great success. In 1960, Drs. John and Rachel Woods, both very competent in Cranio-Sacral manipulation, spent a year at Still-Hildreth Sanatorium studying any possible relationship between cranial dysfunction and mental illness. They found a consistent decrease in the Cranial Rhythmic Impulse (CRI) in the mentally ill. *(81)* The CRI is the very subtle palpable motion in the cranial mechanism which is synchronous with the motion of the brain and fluctuation of the Cerebro-Spinal fluid taking place internally. The normal rate is 10 to 12 cycles a minute. In severe nervous and mental diseases the Woods found rates a slow as 4 to 5 cycles per minute. They also found that such cases respond to Cranial OMT. The brain being such an important organ, nutrition is extremely important.

Urology

Many problems of the kidneys and bladder result from alterations of blood and nerve supply to those organs, and will respond to OMT. Very often problems in the low back and pelvis will cause urinary frequency or urgency in adults, but may result in bed-wetting in children. Checking Chapman's and viscero-somatic reflexes will reveal the presence of infections and more serious problems. These same reflexes will also differentiate appendicitis or ovarian problems. There are few things more painful than a kidney stone. Deep inhibitory pressure over the viscerosomatic reflex from a kidney stone will ease the pain and help pass the stone if it isn't too large.

Obstetrics–Gynecology

There is probably no other area of health care where OMT is of greater benefit than in obstetrics and gynecology. Lets start from the beginning. Women with low back dysfunction are very likely to have low back pain and uterine cramping with their periods. Many will also be unable to conceive unless their back problems are corrected by OMT. Low back problems are also associated with erectile problems in men.

Regular OMT throughout pregnancy will keep the mother more comfortable, improve her chances of having a healthy baby, and make her labor and delivery easier. Osteopaths have been practicing painless childbirth from the very beginning. After delivery two things are very important. The first is to check the mother's pelvis. During the last few weeks of pregnancy, some interesting things take place. The placenta, which is the special organ that develops early in pregnancy, attaches itself to the wall of the uterus and provides the connection between the mothers blood and the developing embryo through the umbilical cord. In this time period, the placenta secretes a special kind of estrogen which relaxes the ligaments of the mother's pelvis to allow for an easier delivery. Another hormone, Relaxin, which the placenta also secretes is thought to help in this regard. Because of this relaxation, the mother's pelvic bones are easily moved, and if they get out of place during the birth process, or in moving the mother following delivery, when the ligaments tighten up the mother is left with some dysfunction. Many women can date low back problems from child-birth, so it is important to check the mother's pelvis at this time. The second very important thing to do is check the baby's head. I mentioned in Chapter 12 of this section, that in the developing baby, the 22 bones which ultimately form the adult skull, are forming from cartilage and membrane, some in 2, 3, or 4 parts. These eventually ossify to form the complete bone, but in this partial state of formation, allow some molding again to make an easier delivery. These bones can be compressed and jammed together during the birth process. The baby's crying at birth is very important. This is commonly thought to bring about the ballooning of the baby's lungs, which it does do, but if the air passages are open, just the ambient air pressure will do that. The crying is create intra-cranial pressure and balloon out the cranial bones so they can develop normally. A depressed baby that doesn't cry, already has some cranial damage, and will suffer more if the problem is not corrected.

The forces which create these problems can be abnormal positioning in the uterus, pressure from another developing fetus, a rapid hard labor which does not allow for gradual molding of the baby's head, a prolonged labor which causes excessive molding, trauma to the mother's abdomen, and often worst of all, the use of forceps or vacuum extraction. Forceps compress the baby's head even when "properly" applied, and vacuum extraction stretches and distorts the baby's head. Both of these procedures should only be used in emergencies.

One of the more severe results of birth trauma is cerebral palsy. About 50 years ago the use of saddle block and outlet forceps became popular in obstetrics. This was often an attempt to make the mother and baby meet the doctor's schedule, rather than letting nature take it's course. Prior to that time the incidence of cerebral palsy was 1 in every 10,000 births, but afterwards became 1 in every 500 births. It took the Medical profession almost 40 years to realize they were injuring thousands of babies with that method. Even in Caesarean Section, because the uterus is a strong muscular organ and requires a certain amount of force to extract the baby, about 10% of these babies show evidence of cranial trauma. *(82)* In some instances the mother has been in labor before the Cesarean surgery is done. Examining the baby's head immediately after birth and correcting the deformities with gentle Osteopathic Cranial technic would prevent most of the serious consequences of birth trauma. In Osteopathic Hospitals where this is practiced this has proven to be true.

Pediatrics

It is a natural sequence to move from obstetrics to pediatrics. Many of the problems in infants that are not immediately apparent are again a result of birth trauma. All too often doctors, both obstetricians and pediatricians, are not aware of this extremely important cranio-sacral concept. When they do recognize a problem, too often they don't have solution for it and they tell the concerned parents, "he or she will outgrow it." Sometimes this does occur because of the body's inherent ability to heal, but tragically sometimes the baby doesn't outgrow it and is left permanently impaired, with cerebral palsy, mental retardation, attention deficit, hyperactivity, perceptual problems, or other handicaps. These could be prevented. Even in genetic problems such as cystic fibrosis, we find significant cranial problems and can give the child some help.

One of the most common problems, but least serious found in infants is colic. This is caused by compression of the base of the baby's skull which we call "condylar compression." The Occipital bone which forms the main part of the base of the skull sits on the first cervical vertebra, the Atlas, on two little rocker like processes which are called condyles. They fit into two elongated saucer-like receptacles on the top of the Atlas which are called facets. These facets deepen and converge anteriorly. The Atlas is well formed at birth, but the Occiput is in four pieces and the compressive force will distort the Occiput and then affect the Vagus nerve which is the major outflow of the Parasympathetic nervous system supplying all of the organs in the chest and abdomen. One of it's functions is to supply the muscles of the stomach which creates the muscular activity which moves the stomach contents on into the small intestine. When over-stimulated, the Vagus causes cramping which can be very painful. This can be relieved by cranial treatment.

Several years ago the daughter of a friend of mine had her first baby while living in Denmark. The baby had terrible colic and was crying day and night. This is very distressing to the infant and the family as well. I talked to the young mother on the phone, and instructed her how to decompress her baby's condylar parts. In 24 hours the baby was nursing and sleeping peacefully. This is not a good thing to do except in emergencies, but it does demonstrate that almost anyone can be taught to do cranio-sacral therapy.

Regurgitation and vomiting are also due to condylar compression. The worse the vomiting, the more severe the baby's head trauma is. Projectile vomiting is a very critical sign, and these cases need immediate Osteopathic cranial care when available.

Another common problem is so-called "congenital torticollis." Torticollis is a musculo-skeletal problem in adults where the head is pulled down to one side by strain to the neck and contraction of the neck muscles on one side, which incidentally responds quickly to OMT. In infants it is much more likely to be due to asymmetry of the Occipital condyles so the head sits on the cervical spine at an angle. It is often complicated by tension in the cervical muscles, but responds to cranial treatment.

Otitis Media, infection of the inner ear, has increased 200% in the last 20 years. The Medical Profession blames some of this on the over-prescribing of anti-biotics. Another factor is more working mothers with their children in Day Care where they are constantly exposed to infections from other children. A study in the Netherlands *(83)* found that children who were not treated for Otitis Media got well just as fast as those who were treated with anti-biotics. They also found that children who had repeated courses of anti-biotics were more apt to have perceptual problems in school, and those who had the ear tubes were likely to have hearing problems. As a result of this study the use of anti-biotics dropped precipitously in the Netherlands. In the United States 98% of doctors still prescribe anti-biotics. Otitis responds to cranial OMT.

One of the most serious consequences of birth trauma is cerebral palsy. More severe cases are immediately apparent and need immediate cranial treatment. One of Dr. Sutherland's (the discoverer of the cranial concept) dreams was to have a cranial Osteopath in every OB Department. This would eliminate most of the problems and handicaps that children suffer. The longer cerebral palsy and other cases of severe birth trauma go, the less that can be done. By the age of six much of the damage becomes permanent, but cranial OMT will still alter their behavior, make them more comfortable, and improve their general health.

As a child gets older, the childhood diseases such as measles, mumps, chicken pox, and others will have a shorter and less complicated recovery with nutrition and careful OMT.

One of the very disturbing problems in children is enuresis or bed-wetting. These children all have low back problems, and many have cranial problems which interfere with the control by higher centers of the basic spinal reflex which empties the bladder when it is full. These cases respond well to OMT.

Another common but ill-defined problem in children is alterations of behavior. Children who are temperamental, rebellious, depressed, aggressive, abusive, withdrawn, etc. all have both nutritional and structural problems. They benefit from improved nutrition and OMT, especially cranial treatment. My father was known internationally as a physician and teacher. He was an outstanding speaker. I had heard him lecture several times while I was in school, and was duly impressed. Shortly after I went into practice with him, he invited me to take part on a program he was putting on for the Kansas Osteopathic Society. I had read that to open a talk you should give an attention getting statement, or something humorous. I searched and read and thought and couldn't come up with any ideas. My father was on the program just before me, and spoke about behavioral problems in children with the recurring theme that when children are misbehaving they should be treated, not punished. He finished, the applause died down, and I was introduced. At last the inspiration came to me, and I said, "I don't like to contradict what my father just told you, but he didn't always practice what he preaches." I don't have any recollection of what I lectured about, but I still remember my opening line. It wasn't the last time my sense of humor got me in trouble.

Dentistry

The teeth are significantly affected by the motion in the cranium, or lack thereof. The most important structures in this regard are the paired maxillary bones which form the upper jaw, and the paired temporal bones. They are in the middle of each side of the skull, contain the hearing mechanism, the organs of equilibrium (the semi-circular canals), and the sockets that the jaw articulates in. Dr. Sutherland referred to the temporal bones as "the trouble makers in the head." The axis of motion of the temporal bone is on an oblique axis about parallel with the external ear canal. The temporal bones can be moved into many abnormal positions by direct trauma to the head or jaw, whip-lash type injuries, stress which can tighten some of the muscles which attach to the bone, postural and occupational habits such as holding the phone on a shoulder, and dental work. Symptoms of such mal-alignments can include headache, tempero-mandibular-joint disease, dizziness (vertigo), ringing or hissing in the ears (tinnitus aurium), mal-occlusion, brain fatigue, facial pain, and visual problems. Many dentists have taken our post-graduate courses in the cranial concept and are members of the Cranial Academy. Some of them feel confident in doing cranial manipulation, others prefer to refer patients to a cranial Osteopath. With significant dental problems it is extremely important to have the two professions work together. Unfortunately, many dentists, like much of the Medical Profession think of the cranium as a solid bony case, and don't understand the bones are moveable. Many patients have had their cranium and enclosed nervous system absolutely ruined by improper dental work done by well-meaning dentists. Later in this chapter I will tell you how to find a dentist who understands this important aspect of dentistry.

Musculo-Skeletal Injuries

Many people think of manipulation only in relation to the musculo-skeletal problems, and indeed it is the most effective way of treating such problems, but as you have seen from the preceding pages, manipulation is effective in all health problems. Musculo-skeletal problems will include all professional and amateur athletes, "weekend warriors," gardeners, accident victims, etc.

One of the most successful basketball coaches of all time, Forest "Phog" Allen of Kansas University, was an Osteopathic Physician and he treated his own players. His book, "My Basketball Bible" *(84)* describes his coaching philosophy, his training methods, and his treatment of his players. Many professional teams, and thousands of Little League, High School and College teams have Osteopathic team physicians. Our Olympic team has a D.O. on the staff.

One of the advantages of Osteopathic Manipulation is that we have a great variety of technics available to suit the particular need of the problem. Recent acute injuries need very gentle technic to reduce swelling, improve circulation, and ease pain. Older chronic problems require more vigorous treatment to improve function.

Many people suffer from bulging or herniated discs (the pads between the vertebrae). X-rays or MRI will reveal the disc problem but don't show the restricted motion of the adjoining vertebrae which put undue pressure on the discs and cause the problem. When vertebral motion is corrected and pressure taken off the disc, most often they will heal. Less than 5% need surgery.

Many State Compensation cases are musculo-skeletal injuries. In 1996 because of problems with our Compensation program here in Colorado, the legislature commissioned a CPA firm, Tillinghast, to do an actuarial analysis of health care providers.

They examined six major health care providers, and found the average cost per patient to be: Osteopaths $953, non-surgical M.D.'s $1304, Surgical M.D.'s $2086, Orthopedists $1118, Mental Health $1607, and Chiropractors $3588. As a result of this studies, Chiropractors were limited in the number of times they could see a State Compensation cases. The same ratio was found in several other states.

Osteopathic Physicians have distinct advantage in musculo-skeletal problems because we have extensive training in diagnosing and treating the musculo-skeletal system, we can "tune in" to what the body is telling us, and when necessary can prescribe medication to counter-act symptoms while we are treating the cause.

Repetitive Motion Syndrome

We have heard a great deal about this condition in recent years. This is a situation where usually a person is in stationary position and goes through repeated motions with their hands, such as computer operators, assembly line workers, filing clerks, etc. The repeated motions cause inflammation of the tendons and ligaments around the wrist. I would prefer to call this condition the "Fixed Position Syndrome." These cases are usually required to be in one spot and build up tension in their upper back and neck which impairs blood and nerve supply to their hands and arms, making them more subject to inflammatory changes. Many of these cases are also nutritionally deficient. The inflammation at the wrist is a result of problems affecting the blood and nerve supply, and responds well to vitamin therapy, heat, and OMT.

Two other conditions which are quite common and have something in common with the Repetitive Motion Syndrome (no doubt that name will stick) are Carpal Tunnel Syndrome and Thoracic Outlet Syndrome. Both of these conditions will have problems in the upper back and base of the neck, the cervico-thoracic area, especially the Thoracic Outlet Syndrome. This is where the blood and nerve supply to the arm and hand comes from. Most cases of both of these conditions have suffered trauma of some kind. Many cases of carpal tunnel have fallen and sprained their wrists. At the same time the force is carried up through the arm and strains the cervico-thoracic area thus impairing the blood and nerve supply and compounding what has happened at the wrist.

The carpal bones form the base of the hand, are in a C shape, and are bridged over by the transverse carpal ligament, thus making a tunnel. Through this tunnel pass the tendons of the muscles of the lower arm which flex the hand and fingers. The tunnel also contains the Median Nerve, one three major nerves which supply the arm and hand. The Median Nerve supplies sensation to the palm of the hand, the palmer surface of the thumb, the index finger, the middle finger, and half of the ring finger. Pressure on that nerve will cause pain, tingling or numbness in the areas just described. If more severe it can affect the ability to approximate the thumb and little finger. Pain above the wrist comes from the origin of the nerve at the cervico-thoracic junction. The other half of the ring finger and the little finger are supplied by the Ulnar Nerve which also arises in the cervico-thoracic area. Benjamin M. Sucher, D.O. of Paradise Valley, Arizona has demonstrated on MRI *(85)* that cases of Carpal Tunnel Syndrome which have not responded to other forms of conservative treatment, will respond to OMT. The MRI's clearly demonstrated enlargement of the damaged carpal tunnel after myo-fascial stretching. Most do not need surgery.

Thoracic Outlet Syndrome is very specifically a problem of the cervico-thoracic area. It frequently is a result of trauma. The person who falls on the shoulder will sprain the cervico-thoracic area, the person who in falling grabs a railing will do the same thing, and very frequently it results from whip-lash type injuries.

Pain or numbness in this instance will be all the way down the arm, not just in the hand, and is most apt to affect the Ulnar nerve causing pain or numbness in the little finger and half of the ring finger. Common Medical treatment is removal of the first rib because the blood and nerve supply come out of the base of the neck, over the first rib, and under the collar bone. This is not always successful in answering the problem, but those who have had such surgery still respond to OMT.

All of these patients need stretching of the cervico-thoracic area in addition to the OMT. I have my patients raise their arms shoulder high with the elbows bent, stretch their arms back, hold them there, take 10 or 12 big deep breaths, and then carefully roll their head in a full circle both clockwise and counterclockwise. This should be repeated several times a day. This stretching exercise is especially important for persons who sit in a fixed position all day.

Preventative Medicine

We are hearing more and more about "preventative medicine." This is a term commonly used when a drug is given to hopefully ward of a certain disease. Preventative medicine is a misnomer. It gives a false sense of security. A drug may prevent a certain disease, but it is very likely to cause other problems, rather than "preventing" disease, a more logical and better goal is to promote wellness. The Kirksville College of Osteopathic Medicine has a wellness program for it's employees, it's staff, it's alumni and their patients. Dr. Still said, "the role of the Osteopath is to find health, anyone can find disease." *(57)*

The best way to promote wellness and preserve health is by following the suggestions for health in Section I, and by getting regular Osteopathic treatment. A periodic "tune-up" is the best way to keep the body functioning properly, to help it cope with stress, and to keep all parts in harmony. The schedule for preventative treatment can vary considerably. It will depend on what you do to help yourself, what you have had in the way of injuries, how much stress you are under, and many other secondary factors. Some patients come in once a week, others once a month, still others one or more times a year.

The Head

I have left this broad category till last, because it is the most important. The greatest contribution to health care since Dr. Still's original Osteopathic concept is Dr. Sutherland's cranial concept. This has provided hope and relief for many conditions for which there had been no effective treatment and not much hope in the past.

We have already discussed some of the importance of cranial treatment in obstetrics, pediatrics, and psychiatry, and now I will include other areas such as eye-ear-nose and throat, endocrinology, and neurology.

One of the most common patient complaints is headache. The International Headache Society lists 178 classifications of headache, the last being "headache not classifiable." Basically there are four mechanisms which produce headache. One that should always be ruled out is pressure from a space-consuming defect such as a tumor, an aneurism (ballooning of an artery) or a hemorrhage. Many times the history and symptoms will be strongly indicative of such a condition, but may require a scan or MRI for confirmation. The three basic physiologic mechanisms which can produce headache are irritation to sensory nerves, congestion, or traction on pain-sensitive structures. Very often there is a combination of these three factors. Irritation to sensory nerves can occur from restrictions of motion in the upper neck affecting nerves which supply the scalp everywhere back of the ears, or problems in the cranial mechanism which can affect the cranial nerves inside the head, primarily the Trigeminal nerve which supply the face and everything inside of the skull. The second, congestion, can be from tension in the neck which blocks the outflow of venous blood from the head. The circulatory system is arranged to provide adequate circulation to the brain, so if venous blockage slows down circulation, the heart pumps harder to force blood to the brain. Or if arteries over-dilate, as in migraine headache, this causes congestion and pressure which can be extremely painful and debilitating. The third is due to traction on pain-sensitive structures inside the head. If enough strain occurs on the cranial bones, the meninges and the major arteries, both of which are pain-sensitive, can be put under tension which will cause pain. As already mentioned, many headaches are combinations of these three mechanisms. Cranial manipulation is the most specific and most effective treatment for such problems. In the event of surgery for the space-consuming defects, gentle cranial treatment can facilitate the patients recuperation.

A common problem, often associated with headache is tinnitus aurium. This may be ringing, hissing, or a blowing sound. This is caused by distortion of the temporal bones, which affects the auditory nerve, or nerve of hearing. Cranial treatment is very effective.

Another common problem is vertigo (dizziness). Many doctors, being unaware of the motion in the cranium, often attribute vertigo to a viral infection, or fluid in the inner ear which there may be as a part of the cranial dysfunction, but this too is caused by alterations of the normal position of the temporal bones. This alters the relationship of the semi-circular canals, which are in the temporal bones, and are the organs of equilibrium. This may also affect the socket the jaw articulates in, causing temperomandibular-joint (TMJ) problems. This is also an important factor in motion sickness. Sometimes vertigo is diagnosed as Meniere's Disease, but this is actually a more severe syndrome which includes vertigo, tinnitus, vomiting, and if not treated, eventually will lead to deafness. This is due to a major distortion of the temporal bones which affects the semi-circular canals, the auditory nerve, the tempero-mandibular joints, and a vomiting center in the brain stem. These problems also respond to cranial treatment, but being a more severe problem, it takes longer.

Whip-lash type injuries often result in headache, vertigo, tinnitus and TMJ dysfunction, and again cranial treatment is by far the most effective treatment.

Many eye problems respond to cranial treatment. One of the first to become noticeable is crossed eyes in infants. This is due to a disturbance of some of the seven bones that make up the orbit, or eye socket, and/or the six small muscles which control eye movement. The earlier treatment is instituted, the better. Nystagmus, or flickering of the eyes will also respond.

In the elderly, cataracts will respond to cranial treatment, improved nutrition, and supplements of vitamin A.

The Pituitary gland, the "master gland," which influences all other endocrine glands is suspended in the middle of the cranium, and can be affected by cranial dysfunction. Thus cranial treatment has much to offer in endocrine imbalances.

Closed head injuries are receiving a great deal of attention nowadays. Such injuries can cause headaches, vertigo, tinnitus, nausea, visual disturbances, loss of memory, disorientation, fatigue, and other symptoms. In more severe ones, sub-dural hemorrhage should be ruled out, which can occur up to three weeks after the injury occurs. One of the persistent problems of closed head injuries can be the cognitive changes, or difficulty in thinking which persists. This can be very disabling. The problem is better recognized now, and psychological tests have been developed to measure the problem, but many doctors, including neurologists, and insurance companies do not understand why it exists. The persistence of the mental difficulty is due to the jamming of the cranial mechanism when the accident occurs. Of course if one is not aware of the cranial mechanism, then one is not in a position to understand the problem. Cranial treatment is by far the most effective approach to such problems. In more severe head and spinal cord injuries, where the patient is a paraplegic or quadriplegic, cranial treatment over a long period of time will keep the patient more comfortable, and help them regain some function.

To cover all of the conditions which can be helped by Osteopathic treatment would require several volumes, but this brief discourse should give the reader some insight as to the possibilities. If any M.D.'s have been brave enough to follow this far, you will have to put aside much that you have been taught, and open your mind to some amazing possibilities.

As I have already mentioned, some Osteopathic Physicians do not do manipulation, many do some OMT, and some of us do a manipulative practice, but can prescribe medication when indicated. When seeking Osteopathic care, you will get the best results from one who does a great deal of OMT because he or she will have developed a better feel of the tissues. If you are seeing a D.O. who does not do OMT, encourage him or her to take some post-graduate courses and add that to their practice. Both of you will benefit from it. The American Academy of Osteopathy and the Kirksville College of Osteopathic Medicine both conduct regular graduate seminars to help D.O.'s improve their manipulative skills in treating all health problems. If you don't have an Osteopath, there are several ways to get a referral. In many instances, the State Osteopathic Society, listed in the phone book, can tell you who in your locality does OMT. A better reference would be the American Academy of Osteopathy. Their website is:

http://www.academyofosteopathy.org

If you don't have a computer (not every one does!), send a self-addressed stamped envelope to:

The American Academy of Osteopathy
3500 De Pauw Blvd. Suite 1080
Indianapolis, IN 46268

For specialists in cranio-sacral treatment, send a self-addressed stamped envelope to:

The Cranial Academy
8202 Clearvista Parkway, #9
Indianapolis, IN 46256

This is also the source of information for dentists who are trained in the cranial concept. Should you have questions, any Osteopath will be glad to answer them.

For problems with severely handicapped children, there is a very special internationally known clinic in San Diego, California, "Osteopathy's Promise to Children." The director is Viola Frymann, D.O., F.A.A.O. Dr. Frymann was a pupil of Dr. Sutherland's, and because she had lost a child of her own to birth trauma, has devoted her life to helping other mothers avoid the grief she suffered. Dr. Frymann is internationally recognized as the leading authority in her field. I have known and worked with Dr. Frymann for 50 years, and she is a legend in her own time. You may contact this clinic in several ways.

Address : Osteopathy's Promise to Children
4135 54th Place, San Diego, CA. 92105
Website: www.osteopathic-ctr-4child.org
E-mail: opc@quik.com
Phone: 619-583-0186

14

Advice

I t might seem that this subject would logically come in
sequence in Section One of structuring one's life to attain
better health. However, in order for the reader to better understand the importance of natural and more conservative approaches
to healthcare, it is important to know more about the structure-
function relationship of the human body, it's innate ability to heal
under many circumstances, and the contribution that Osteopathic
manipulative treatment can offer in this regard, so I have placed
this chapter here in section II.

Advice is defined as "A recommendation regarding a decision or course of conduct." *(86)* There is all kinds of advice on
every subject imaginable. Some advice can be helpful and beneficial, but some can be dangerous and harmful. Advice on in-
vestments can be risky at times, but advice on health problems
can be even riskier and have dire consequences when wrong.
How can you tell good advice from bad? You can't always, but
there are some things you need to keep in mind. First of all consider the source. Your in-laws and your hair-dresser or your bar-
tender may have your best interest at heart, but may not be well-
informed. What are the credentials of the person offering the advice? This of course can be risky, too. Some apparently well-

educated persons are very narrow-minded and lacking in correct information. Does the advice come from a special interest group? Is there some financial incentive to give certain advice? Above all always use common sense, keeping in mind your track record in having common sense.

Let's start with nutrition. Probably the most common advice for nutrition is "eat a balanced diet." That should immediately tell you that your advisor knows little about adequate nutrition. What is a "balanced diet ?" It usually means get the three food groups, fat, carbohydrate and protein. Following that you probably still won't get enough protein. And if you have specific vitamin or mineral deficiencies, it won't answer the problem unless you supplement those nutrients. This was discussed in chapter one of section one. Unfortunately, many dieticians are of the "balanced diet" persuasion. A competent nutritionist is a much better source. Again unfortunately, many doctors are a poor source of correct information. In many instances your healthfood store manager is more knowledgeable, but if you have a significant health problem, find a holistic doctor to advise you.

One of the worst sources of helpful advice is our own government. The Department of Agriculture puts out some helpful information at times, but too often is off base. Other government agencies with some jurisdiction over our health suffer from the same lack of knowledge. All too often their advice comes from the traditional medical perspective and it's addiction to drug therapy.

The worst example of the government's concern for our health and their advice in that regard, is the Surgeon General's warning on cigarettes that it may be "harmful to your health." Over 400,000 deaths a year from smoking, and over 70 billion in cost is indeed harmful. Then on the other hand the government continues to make attempts to limit the number of vitamins you can take, and attempts to control their availability. Good nutrition saves thousands of lives every year, and there is no way of calculating the expense it saves by healing sickness and preventing degenerative diseases. Because nutrition is now big business, the government is trying to bring nutritional supplements under the control of the Food and Drug Administration. This would be an enormous mistake, and would further damage our poor state of health. A recent survey by the World Health Organization *(87)* of the level of health in 141 organized countries in the world, found that the United States ranked 37th, even though we spend the most on health care of all those countries.

The government and many doctors warn against taking vitamin supplements, but reactions are very rare. Several years ago there were several deaths among infants and children from taking their mother's supplements. Investigation showed they had taken ferrous sulfate, an inorganic iron supplement, which destroys vitamin E in the system and is known to be toxic. Identifying the problem put an end to it. Natural supplements contain an organic source of iron which is non toxic, but can still be a problem with rare individuals suffering from hemosiderosis, where they store large amounts of iron.

Some people get allergic reactions to vitamin supplements, which may be a reaction either to some of the ingredients or to the binder which holds the tablet together. There are non-allergenic supplements available which can avoid those problems. A few people get an upset stomach from vitamin supplements. Supplements are concentrated and should be taken with meals to dilute them, and it is at that time your metabolism needs the vitamins and minerals. Also avoiding food intolerances as described in "Eat Right 4 Your type" can improve your utilization of the right supplement.

The Food and Drug Administration (FDA) is one of the worst sources of advice on good health, something they are supposed to be promoting. What they are promoting is the use of a growing list of drugs, all of which have side-effects, many of them fatal. The FDA is a powerful, political regulatory agency, steeped in traditional medicine which changes very slowly, and appears to be strongly influenced by the rich, powerful pharmaceutical industry. The FDA regulates all drugs and health-related products. While it is important to keep obviously harmful products off the market, the main function of the FDA is to approve new drugs that have been developed by the pharmaceutical industry. Physicians Desk Reference *(88)* which lists all prescription drugs, does not say how many prescription drugs there are, but does list 3,600 specific reactions to drugs, and lists the American equivalent of 15,000 foreign medications. You can hardly find a page in PDR that doesn't list fatal reactions. Typically if a drug shows some improvement in 60 - 70% of cases, 20 - 30% showing no improvement, 10 - 15 % being worse, and only 1 - 2% showing fatal reactions, it is considered a good drug. I would point out again that over 160.000 persons a year die from drug reactions in the United States.

The FDA's favoritism for the pharmaceutical industry can be illustrated by an example published by Dr. Robert Atkins in his "Health Revelations" *(89)* wherein the FDA banned the import of red yeast from China which contains cholestin, a natural supplement which lowers the amount of LDL or "bad" cholesterol. Cholestin costs about $20 - $30 a month, while drugs which produce the same lowering effect, but always with the possibility of side-effects, cost about $120 - $300 per month. The case was reversed by a U.S. District Court.

The pharmaceutical industry is rich and powerful. It has grown because of traditional medicine's philosophy of prescribing a pill or shot for every symptom that presents itself for man and animal. It is fostered by massive advertising campaigns promoting taking a pill for every little thing, which is not good advice. Then when side-effects occur, which is frequently the case, another pill is given to counter-act the side-effect. It is not unusual to see patients on 7, 8 or more medications, and most often they act like zombies. Many of these drugs cause new problems and the list of "iatrogenic" or doctor-caused diseases is growing every year. Large sums are spent on research to find new drugs, additional amounts are spent to test the efficacy of these drugs to the satisfaction of the FDA, and at present these costs are over 8 billion dollars a year! Drug companies say this is why prescriptions cost so much, but this not the whole story. Drug companies spend more than that 8 billion promoting their products. They spend great amounts in media advertising, and additional amounts supporting medical magazines which are sent to doctors whether they want them or not. They employ pharmaceutical representatives which visit doctors offices, hospitals, and clinics promoting their products and handing out free samples. Drug companies do extensive entertaining of doctors at regional and national Osteopathic and Medical meetings. They provide gifts for doctors, and underwrite trips to exotic places for medical meetings. And who pays for all this? You and insurance companies who pay for prescriptions. Pharmaceutical companies can advertise the "healing effects" of their drugs, but natural food supplement manufacturers cannot make the same claims. Does this make sense?

Some pharmaceutical companies market vitamin products. Chemists have been able to synthesize some vitamins, so they are the same as the natural product, but the significant difference is in the completeness of the products. The typical pharmaceutical "B complex" contains 4 or 5 synthetic B vitamins, whereas the natural product contains 11 components. When both parties advise you to use their product, whose advice are you going to take? Some nutritionists say if you take some of the B vitamins and are deficient in others you can accentuate the deficiency of those you are not getting. The same is true of Vitamin C. The drug store product is usually just ascorbic acid, while the natural product contains ascorbic acid, hesperidin, bioflavonoids, and rutin, all of which your body needs. Whose advice are you going to take?

There is no question that some drugs are helpful and at times save lives, but unfortunately they often take lives, which is accepted as part of the practice of medicine. Most drugs just counteract symptoms, and they are classified as such, for example, antibiotics, anti-inflammatories, anti-arthritics, anti-coagulants, anticonvulsants, anti-depressants, anti-diabetics, anti-diuretics, antifungals, anti-histamines, anti-hypertensives. Because most drugs just counter-act symptoms, and it is still up to the body's various defense mechanisms to over-come the problem, why not take a natural approach and support the body's defenses in the first place? This approach is why nutritional supplements, herbs, Osteopathy, Naturopathy, acupuncture, and many other "alternative" methods are growing in popularity.

One of the sources of advice I find most objectionable is the typical medical advice column in most newspapers. All too often the advice falls in the usual toxic, invasive practice of traditional medicine. For instance the use of aspirin for fevers. Fever is the body's natural response to an infection, and unless it gets too high, 104 in children and 102 in adults, it should be allowed to run it's course. In an infection when there is no fever response, hot baths should be used to elevate body temperature and help nature eradicate the infection. One medical column recommended aspirin to prevent colon-rectal cancer. Proper diet has been shown to dramatically reduce colon cancer. Aspirin is widely recommended to prevent heart attacks. Again, proper diet will dramatically reduce all forms of heart disease. Over 5,000 people a year die from taking aspirin, does it make sense to take it as a "preventative?"

A letter to a medical column asked about depression. The typical response, "take anti-depressants," all of which have a long list of side-effects, including fatal reactions. Some of these deaths are from reactions to the drug, others have been suicide. Most cases of depression respond well and safely to vitamin B complex which supports the nervous system, St. Johns wart which has natural anti-depressant effects, and Osteopathic treatment, especially cranial treatment which improves the function of the brain and nervous system.

Another writer complained that her doctor put her on muscle relaxants for acute low back pain which hadn't cleared up in several weeks, so she went to a chiropractor and after several treatments she was better. She wondered why her doctor didn't refer her to a chiropractor in the first place. The medical expert replied "that many doctors do not realize the benefits of spinal manipulative therapy." He went on to say that "this type of treatment can be beneficial for soft tissue injuries, and should be an option for patients where serious under-lying pain has been ruled out." This demonstrates some of the short-comings of both the chiropractic and medical professions, and why an Osteopathic Physician who does manipulation is the best choice. As outlined in Chapter 9, Chiropractic was "discovered" in 1893 after D.D. Palmer spent two weeks in Kirksville where he was treated by Dr. Still. Palmer picked up just a few rudimentary technics from Dr. Still, but enough to establish a reputation for healing. Chiropractors have increased their knowledge through the years, but still don't understand all of the intricacies of the musculo-skeletal system, and therefore at times are not able to treat more complicated problems appropriately. We who do Osteopathic manipulation as a specialty, consistently see patients who have been under repeated chiropractic adjustments and are no better, or sometimes worse. Also, Chiropractors do not have medical training, and therefore in some instances do not recognize under-lying medical problems where adjustments are contra-indicated. Incidents are abundant where Chiropractors have treated cancer and other serious pain-producing illnesses, with dire consequences. Osteopathic Physicians have complete medical training, plus their complete manipulative training, and are thus able to do a differential diagnosis in serious cases. They also have the knowledge and training to effectively treat more than "soft tissue" injuries. Medical doctors do not get any manipulative training in Medical School, but many have taken post-graduate training in manipulation which they call "manual medicine." Recognizing their deficiency, the American Medical Association has appointed a task force to investigate including manipulation or "manual medicine" in medical school curriculum. Increasing awareness of the importance of the musculo-skeletal system as a source of many problems has prompted more M.D.'s to refer patients for physical therapy, and some will refer patients to Chiropractors for musculo-skeletal problems. Not many will refer to Osteopathic Physicians (D.O.'s) however because we are greater competition to them because we also practice medicine. This is one of the outstanding things about Andrew Weil, M.D. the so-called "guru of holistic medicine," who having observed some of the things that Osteopathy has to offer, actively promotes Osteopathy in his health newsletter.

Another writer asked about macular degeneration. The writer of the medical column responded that "a treatment is not available." This is not entirely true. Our tissues are very highly developed, and we do not have the regenerative powers that lower forms of life have, but many "incurable" diseases such as macular degeneration, if caught early enough will respond to a rigid nutritional program and Osteopathic treatment. Of special importance in macular degeneration are vitamins A and E, and cessation of smoking.

Another writer complained that her 75 year old mother was being treated with anti-biotics for dizziness. The expert stated that "vertigo (dizziness) is often a medical enigma." It needn't be. Most cases of vertigo are caused by alterations of the cranial mechanism, especially the temporal bone which holds the hearing mechanism and the semi-circular canals, which are the organs of equilibrium, as explained in Chapter 13. Many doctors, not knowing about the cranial motion, pass off vertigo as a viral infection, or fluid in the inner ear. This lady's treating doctor probably thought her problem was due to an infection and so prescribed an anti-biotic, but it is well known that anti-biotics are not effective against viruses. The expert went on to recommend an examination by an ear, nose and throat specialist, as well as a neurologist. This would of course involve laboratory tests, scans, and MRI's at considerable expense. A good cranial Osteopath would have been able to make a good diagnosis, determine if something more serious was involved, and given the lady relief from her symptoms at a fraction of the cost.

Another writer asked about Attention Deficit Disease. Again the answer of "no known cure, but symptoms are helped by Ritalin." This is a widely used but very controversial treatment because of the many adverse effects that Ritalin can have. A much better answer is Osteopathic cranial treatment. Nearly all cases of A.D.D. can be traced to birth trauma. There are thousands of such cases, and it is tragic that the medical profession and the public in general doesn't know that there is a gentle, natural way to remove the cause of the symptoms, and not just give a drug to counter-act the symptoms.

A writer asked about severe acne in her teenage daughter. This is a very common problem in which the oil glands of the skin get clogged, and then become infected. The response, "take her to a dermatologist and get her on oral anti-biotics." This is the common answer, but anti-biotics don't always bring about a remission of the infection, and they destroy the normal bacteria of the intestinal tract which produce natural vitamin B complex, and vitamin K. Acne can nearly always be controlled by nutritional changes. Teenage girls are notorious for eating poorly. They should avoid all sugars (which favor infections), refined starch, fat-saturated starch (such as french fries and donuts). They need adequate protein intake, a good multivitamin, additional vitamins A and B complex which are important for the skin, unsaturated fatty acids found in vegetable oils to help metabolize oils and fats, and lecithin also to help metabolize the oils and fats. Large doses of vitamin C, without which our immune systems cannot function, will help clear up the infection.

Another writer to an advice column asked about neck pain that radiated to his hand. He said his family doctor said it was a muscle strain. The problem may have started with a strain, but no muscle runs the full length of the arm, so it has to be a sensory nerve involvement coming from the neck. The "expert" responded that it was "a radiculopathy usually caused by a bulging disc." He recommended that an X-ray should be done, or better still an MRI, and see a neurologist. The vast majority of such problems are due to dysfunction of the vertebrae in the lower part of the neck, which affect the nerves to the arm and hand. A good Osteopath could quickly diagnose the problem, usually without the expense of an X-ray at $100 to $125, or an MRI at around $1000. If the problem were more serious with some disc involvement, the majority of these respond to careful manipulation, and most do not need disc surgery.

Another writer asked about osteo-arthritis of the knees. The answer was to take Vitamin D. Vitamin D has a small role in arthritis. Of much greater help is glucosamine sulfate or chondroitin sulfate both of which are precursors of human cartilage, and over a period of time will help healing in the cartilage of joints. Vitamin A in doses of 75,000 to 100,000 units a day will help heal the synovial membrane which lines joints, and vitamin C will help reduce the inflammation. A high protein diet will also provide necessary healing substances. Osteo-arthritis is an inflammatory condition of joints which can be caused by trauma, over-usage or poor nutrition, or a combination of those factors.

Infants are always a matter of concern, and a writer asked about the use of the open-topped helmet for infants to correct the positional plagiocephaly (distortion of the head) that may result from having babies sleep on their backs to prevent the sudden infant death syndrome. SIDS can be a result of babies sleeping face down and suffocating. The helmets cost in the neighborhood of $3,000. On the surface the reshaping of the baby's head looks good, but the helmets are stiff and impersonal. They will leave areas of restricted motion in the baby's cranial mechanism which may lead to problems later in life, such as visual problems requiring glasses, or tempero-mandibular joint problems, or headaches. A much more rational, gentle and economical answer is gentle Osteopathic cranial treatment which leaves the cranial mechanism in much better over-all functional capability.

Another writer asked about prostatitis, which is a bothersome inflammation or infection of the prostate gland in males, which causes many problems with urination and sexual function. The response was anti-biotic therapy, hot sitz baths, lots of fluids, and a "well balanced diet." All too often anti-biotics are ineffective against todays infective organisms. Hot sitz baths to increase circulation do help, and drinking fluids to flush out the urinary tract do help. More specific are large doses of vitamin C which support the immune system, and by acidifying the urine helps the body overcome the infection. Osteopathic treatment to improve blood and nerve supply is also effective.

These are just a few examples of the many common problems which have more natural, more effective, and usually less expensive solutions than are offered by traditional medicine.

There is all kinds of advice on nutrition, much of it confusing and contradictory. I find two excellent sources of reliable information to be Dr. Robert Atkin's "Health Revelations" published by Agora Health Publications, 105 West Monument Street, Baltimore, Maryland 21201, and Dr. William Campbell Douglas's "Second Opinion," published by Second Opinion Publishers, Inc. 7100 Peach-tree Dunwoody Road, Suite 7100, Atlanta, Georgia 30328. Both of these gentlemen are medical doctors, who take a strong stand for natural remedies, use common sense, and reveal many of the failings of traditional medicine. They must not be very popular in medical circles, but they are doing a world of good.

One of my pet peeves is in regard to fever, and this is a serious sources of poor advice. Fever is the body's natural response to an infection. In the presence of an infection, if the body does not respond with a fever, it shows the immune system is not functioning properly. Many doctors treat fever merely as a symptom, and prescribe an anti-pyretic (fever reducer) such as aspirin, tylenol, or ibuprofen. They are taught to do this in Medical School. And there are massive advertising campaigns promoting anti-pyretics for every fever. This is a big mistake. Anti-pyretics not only reduce fever, they also oxidize vitamin C which is very important to fight infections. Fever may be localized as in an abscess, or it may be generalized as in flu or other systemic infections. Aulus Cornelius Celsus, 25 BC - 50 AD, a Roman Patrician and medical writer provided the classic description of inflammation. "Rubor et tumor, cum calor et dolor." Redness and swelling, with fever and pain. *(90)* The level of the fever is of prime importance. Most children can tolerate a fever of 104 unless they are prone to seizure activity. Most adults can tolerate a fever of 103. When fevers reach this point, then measures should be taken to control them. In the presence of infectious conditions where there is no fever response, hot baths or other sources of heat should be given to increase the fever and aid the body's immune system. A number of years ago, a French M.D., winner of the Nobel Prize in Medicine, visited this country for the first time and was appalled at the use of aspirin for fever. About the same time a prominent M.D. here in Denver retired, and was honored by the Medical Society. In his remarks the doctor stated he had come to Colorado during the flu epidemic of 1917-18 and was told to treat it with cough syrup and aspirin, which he did, but stated he lost many patients.

Patients with fever should be treated with adequate fluid intake, large doses of vitamin C, some easily digested form of protein such as broth or light soup. Infants can be given vitamin C dissolved in water or fruit juice. Adelle Davis *(2)* said infants with severe infections can be given 1000 mg. per hour around the clock. This is important because the body cannot manufacture white blood cells, one of the most important lines of defense, without Vitamin C. Older children can use the chewable vitamin C tablets and often like the tart taste. The use of chicken soup by the Jewish community is legendary, and has been the subject of many jokes, but this has a firm basis in reality. It provides both liquid and light protein to support metabolism and the immune system. Acute infections of all kinds respond beautifully to Osteopathic treatment of one kind or another. Flu, colds, pneumonia, sinusitis, colitis, cystitis, otitis media, mumps, whatever, all respond to gentle Osteopathic treatment of various kinds. Such treatment eases the patients discomfort, encourages circulation, improves elimination of waste products, enhances the immune system, and establishes a good rapport with the patient which is important especially in serious diseases. There is great concern in the medical community about the very virulent strains of bacteria and viruses that are being produced, and that they have nothing to combat them with. They continue to over-look the body's own immune system and how it can be supported.

The internet has rapidly become a source of information and advice. Even prescription drugs have become available, which is not good. They are "controlled substances" for good reason. As yet there are few controls in this area, so choose carefully. There are many test kits of various kinds, and many "Health Aids." Be careful and use common sense!

More and more advertising and advice for health care are being direct-mailed. I received an ad for a "super" co-enzyme Q-10 which supposedly made it more digestible. It said, "just try to dissolve your co-enzyme Q-10 in water." Common sense would tell you that unless you had just drunk a copious amount of water, your normal stomach content would not be just water. Stomach content is normally acid, and then in the small intestine are digestive enzymes to carry on the digestion.

Arthritis affects over 60 million Americans. It is the #1 health problem in persons over 50 years of age. It accounts for over 80 million doctor visits per year, and millions of hospitalizations at great cost, which amounts to about 20% of our Gross National Product. I have already discussed in Chapter One of Section I how Dale Alexander in his Book, "Arthritis and Common Sense" *(12)* gave some good advice based on a false premise, and what the Medical response was. That attitude still exists. In the May-June issue of "Arthritis Today," *(91)* their senior editor in response to a question from a reader about "The Arthritis Cure" by Jason Theodosakis, MD, came down hard and unreasonably on Dr. Theodosakis. The editor said, "where the authors advice goes against medical wisdom, as well as my own sense of ethics in his strong promotion of nutritional supplements. The cornerstone of the doctor's 'cure' is in the use of two unproven remedies: glucosamine sulfate and chondroitin sulfate." Medical wisdom? That is reminiscent of George Carlin's famous monologue about "military intelligence!" The whole history of medicine has been one of rejection of new ideas, which in time have proven to be of great benefit. This is true of Semmelweis and his antisepsis; Koch, Pasteur, and Jenner and vaccination; Hahnemann and homeopathy; and Still and Osteopathy. And "his own sense of ethics?" Isn't it more ethical to search for ways to help suffering mankind, than to stay in the same old rut of ineffective, toxic medicines? In 1958 the National Osteopathic Convention was in Washington , D.C. This is a time I will never forget because Dwight Eisenhower was President, and he was a patient of my father's. I had treated Mrs. Eisenhower, and while at the Convention, she showed me and my wife through the White House. That was a great thrill, and was a time when being in the White House really meant something. One of the lectures at the convention was an official of the National Health Institute, talking about what a problem arthritis was. The early anti-inflammatories were in use, and he said they masked symptoms, but allowed the disease to progress. He said they didn't know what to do about it. The article in "Arthritis Today" goes on to say that natural remedies can be dangerous, citing the problem in the late 80's when a number of people became ill from taking L-tryptophan, a natural sleep aid. That problem was traced to a contaminated batch of tryptophan from Japan, and had nothing to do with the tryptophan itself, but it has never been brought back on the market. But dangerous? Over 160,000 people a year die from prescription drugs! Isn't that dangerous? Both glucosamine sulfate and chondroitin sulfate have proven to be very beneficial in arthritis, especially when combined with other nutritional changes.

At this point you may be wondering about the advice I am giving. Is this author a reliable source of advice? My advice is based on 50 years of successful Osteopathic practice, extensive reading, thousands of hours of post-graduate education, both listening and lecturing, and a good dose of common sense. My advice is not going to solve everyone's problems, but it will be a good start. The important thing to remember is to take charge of your life and do the right things. Be the Master of your Fate, and the Captain of your Soul!

15

What the Future Holds

O steopathy has weathered many storms, and will undoubtedly face many more. There have been those who have predicted the demise of Osteopathy, and some still do, but we are still here. Many years ago Dr. Still said, "The greatest threat to our profession will come from within." *(67)* His final words on this earth were, "keep it pure, boys, keep it pure." Those of us who have kept it pure are in the minority. Some of the Osteopathic Profession want to be considered part of mainstream medicine, and indeed they are, in spite of the efficacy of Osteopathic treatment, and in spite of the growing demand for "alternative medicine," Osteopathy being the best. One of my reasons for writing this book was to inform more of the public about what real Osteopathy is. The American Osteopathic Association (A.O.A.) has done a poor job in their public relations in this regard. Two years ago, in response to pressure from Osteopathic students that Osteopathy is not well-enough known, the A.O.A. launched the "Unity Campaign." It's purpose was to unify the profession, to make the term "D.O." a household word, and publicize the difference between a D.O. and an M.D. The theme of the Unity Campaign is that Osteopathic Physicians "treat the whole body," whereas M.D.'s focus on symptoms, one body part, or one organ system. The Osteopathic Profession has always claimed to be a separate and distinct form of Medicine. Treating the whole body, for true Osteopaths, is simply putting into practice the basic philosophy of considering the whole body as an inter-related complex of all it's parts and organ systems. However, the important difference is that true Osteopaths do some form of manipulation as discussed in previous chapters in this section. The use of O.M.T. is what has made Osteopathy, and it's modern counter-part, Osteopathic Medicine, so successful, and gained world-wide recognition. But here is the catch. Because some Osteopathic Physicians do not do O.M.T., the A.O.A. cannot promote that aspect of Osteopathic Medicine as an aspect of our distinction, so the Unity Campaign is less than a half truth. In 1999 I wrote to 10 of the leaders of our profession, the President, President-elect, Past-President, Speaker of the House, Director of Education, etc. discussing this great discrepancy, and not one of them responded to my letter. In addition to educating the public about what a D.O is, and what it should be, the American Osteopathic Association should be encouraging it's members to adhere to Dr. Still's teachings. They should be stressing it's efficacy and cost-effectiveness in today's cost-conscious managed care. Of course this is a complicated problem. All D.O.'s receive significant training in O.M.T. while in school. Some learn just enough to pass their tests, and then let it drop. Others learn it, and start using it, but when they get in to the clinical years of their training, if they are in situations where they don't see O.M.T. being used, they lose interest in doing it, and it takes a lot of time to develop skills in doing O.M.T.. Many students though, learn O.M.T., grasp it's significance, and make a point of increasing their knowledge and skill. Many of such motivated students attend the annual meeting of the American Academy of Osteopathy held each March. Here they get advanced training, and "hands-on" experience with the best in the Osteopathic Profession.

One of the major problems in maintaining interest in and

developing skills in manipulation with students is when they graduate and go into their internships and residencies. We graduate more Osteopathic students than we have intern and resident slots for them, so some have to take Allopathic internships and residencies where they don't see O.M.T. utilized, and in some Osteopathic internships and residencies they don't see that much being used. This has been recognized as a problem for many years, and the A.O.A. keeps talking about making O.M.T. training mandatory in all internships and residencies, but as yet they haven't. Again as part of the Unity Campaign the A.O.A. is talking about this requirement, but we will see if it is ever done. The American Academy of Osteopathy has the qualified people to accomplish this important task if called upon. This is the most important part of Osteopathic post-graduate education, but is sadly neglected in many instances.

Both the American Osteopathic Association (A.O.A.) and the American Medical Association (A.M.A.) have had programs of Continuing Medical Education (C.M.E.) to keep doctors aware of new developments, to review present knowledge, and have required it to maintain membership in their respective organizations. The A.M.A. discontinued their C.M.E. Program because less than 50% of M.D.'s were members of the A.M.A. The A.O.A. has maintained their C.M.E. program, and more than 75% of D.O.'s belong to the A.O.A. We are required to take 150 hours of designated C.M.E. courses every three years, and those of us who are certified must take an additional 50 hours of C.M.E. relating to our specialty. This is a well-intentioned program aimed at keeping doctors from "getting in a rut," but it is badly abused. I served on the A.O.A. C.M.E. Committee for five years. According to A.O.A. C.M.E. regulations, accredited C.M.E. Programs must have O.M.T. integrated into the program. This was never enforced when I was on the Committee. In order to get credit one is expected to attend meetings of course. This is also not enforced. One of the major violations occurs at the national A.O.A. Convention. The opening day if you sign a card and turn it in, you are automatically credited with attendance for the whole five days and 25 hours C.M.E. credit. My State Association, The Colorado Society of Osteopathic Medicine, has a popular Ski-C.M.E. Program every February at Keystone Ski Resort. Lectures are scheduled from 6 to 9 in the morning and 4 to 6 in the afternoon so the days are free to ski. There will typically be 200 to 300 registered, but when you attend a lecture there will be a fraction of that number in attendance, but everyone gets the 40 hours of C.M.E. credit. It would require a great deal more paper-work to monitor each registrant's attendance at lectures, but there is really no point in having regulations that are automatically broken and ignored. The situation is quite different at meetings of the American Academy of Osteopathy and The Cranial Academy. Everyone is there to learn more Osteopathy and they attend all meetings. As I mentioned earlier, many students who recognize the importance of the Osteopathic concept, attend these meetings, some on scholarship, others at their own expense.

In June of 2000 a conference was held by the A.O.A. Educational Policies and Procedures Review Committee to determine if the Osteopathic Profession is indeed a distinct and separate School of Medicine, and if it is, can it remain so. The Committee felt that the distinction between the Osteopathic Medical Profession and the Allopathic Profession has decreased some by some Osteopaths becoming more Allopathically oriented, and some M.D.'s becoming more holistically oriented. Some felt the two professions will eventually merge, others did not. One member of the Committee, a former President of the A.O.A. said, "They (the A.M.A.) will adopt the best we have to offer, as we will ideally adopt the best they have to offer." *(92)* This states two absolutely opposing ideas. Dr. Still's idea was to "improve the practice of medicine, surgery and obstetrics" by substituting manipulative procedures for much of traditional medicine. This would mean M.D.'s adopting the best we have to offer. If Medical

Schools do include "Manual Medicine" in the curriculum, that will be a big step in the right direction, but it will be focused on just musculo-skeletal problems and it will be generations, if ever, that they understand the whole Osteopathic philosophy of the complete structure-function relationship as described in Chapter 8 of this section. In the meantime, one of the biggest problems and failures of Osteopathic Medicine has been "adopting the best they have to offer," practicing Medicine instead of Osteopathy. I distinguish between those two differences in our own profession by the terms "Osteopathic Medicine" and Osteopathy. It is my firm belief that those of us who practice Osteopathy, particularly the members of the American Academy of Osteopathy, and the Cranial Academy will do everything possible to maintain a separate and distinct Osteopathic Profession.

The distinction between Osteopathic Medicine and Allopathic Medicine will be further diluted by what Andrew Weil, M.D. calls Integrative Medicine *(93)*, "which combines the best ideas and practices of alternative and conventional medicine in order to maximize the body's innate potential for self-healing."

More and more healthcare providers, physical therapists and "body workers" of all kinds, are using manipulative procedures with varying degrees of success. All major manipulative procedures in use have originated with the Osteopathic Profession. We are recognized world-wide as the best in this regard, and it will be up to us to remain so.

Chiropractic was "discovered" after D.D. Palmer, a "magnetic healer" from Davenport, Iowa who spent two weeks with Dr. Still in Kirksville in 1893, a year after Dr. Still had opened his first Osteopathic College. They have taken a different turn, and with lesser educational requirements are more numerous than Osteopaths. Chiropractors claim they are the only ones that are taught and are qualified to do manipulation. This is totally false. There are 45,000 Osteopathic Physicians who have been taught to do Manipulation, but some do not use it, as we have discussed.

There are thousands of M.D.'s who have been taught to do manipulation which they call "manual medicine," most of whom are members of the International Federation of Manual Medicine and the North American Federation of Manual Medicine. Many D.O.'s also belong to these two organizations. In the mid 1900's John N. Mennell, M.D. from England was world- famous for his skill in manipulation.

In late 2000 the American Chiropractic Association brought suit against the U. S. Department of Health and Human Services (H.H.S.) alleging the following:

(1) "The Health Care Finance Administration (H.C.F.A.) has failed to provide Medicare+ Choice beneficiaries access to chiropractic services as required by statute - evidence is a study done by the Office of the Inspector General that indicates that Medicare fee for service had more chiropractic services than under Medicare+ Choice.

(2) Physical Therapists cannot perform spinal manipulation of the spine as they do not meet the definition of "physician" under Medicare and, as such, spinal manipulation by a P.T. is not a Medicare covered service.

(3) Medical Doctors and Osteopathic Physicians are not educated or trained to perform manual manipulation of the spine to correct subluxation, a unique service limited to chiropractors in many states.

(4) Because MD's and DO's do not refer patients to chiropractors, and because there is prejudice against chiropractors by the medical community, all Medicare managed care plans must either allow self-referrals for manual manipulation of the spine to correct a subluxation by a chiropractor or must include one or more chiropractors on the staff or panel of the plan to operate as a chiropractic gatekeeper.

(5) Medicare has misspent beneficiary funds by paying for non-chiropractic manual manipulation of the spine to correct a subluxation."

The matter will be decided in the courts, but it does sound a little paranoid. I would make some comments though. Physical therapists can and do spinal manipulation, but are not eligible for Medicare reimbursement because they are not physicians. However, they have their own C.P.T. codes and can be reimbursed. Following the dictionary definition of "physician," *(94)* "a doctor or person who has been educated, trained and licensed to practice the art and science of medicine." Therefore chiropractors are also not physicians, but are "doctors of chiropractic."

Medical doctors and Osteopaths are very definitely educated and trained to perform manual manipulation of the spine, as previously discussed, and all other portions of the musculo-skeletal system. However we treat "somatic dysfunctions" of the musculo-skeletal system. Chiropractors are taught to "adjust" subluxations of the spine, which are defined as "partial dislocations of the spine." *(ibid)* There is a significant difference in these two approaches. The complexities of somatic dysfunctions of the spine, and their far-reaching effects on both the voluntary and involuntary nervous systems, and the circulatory systems are only completely understood by Osteopaths.

In item 4, there may be good reason why M.D.'s and D.O.'s don't refer to chiropractors as a general rule.

Medicare funds for manipulation of the spine by D.O.'s and M.D.'s is very appropriate, and chiropractors should be reimbursed for only adjustments of subluxations.

Chiropractors make inroads by lawsuits such as this. Many insurance companies will make concessions just to avoid costly litigation. In this instance, the Department of Health and Human Services is choosing to settle the matter in court.

Speaking of insurance companies, they are becoming an ever-increasing problem. There was a time when insurance covered hospitalization and injuries from accidents. As time passed, people demanded more and more coverage, so insurance companies added more coverage, but increased premiums to cover the cost. There are always people who try to take advantage of the situation, and there are always a few unscrupulous doctors, clinics, and laboratories who indulge in fraudulent activities, so insurance companies tighten their restrictions and make it difficult for everyone. There are more forms to fill out, the forms are more complicated, and there are more letters to write. Along the way "second opinion" was instituted, primarily to cut down on unnecessary surgeries, but studies showed it made no difference. Then "independent medical examinations" (I.M.E.) were instituted by insurance companies. They seem to feel that a physician who spends 30 minutes with a patient knows more about them than the physician who has followed the patient's problems for several months. Insurance companies will pay $600 for an I.M.E., and quickly authorize $1000 for an M.R.I., but refuse to pay for treatment that has been helping the patient. Insurance companies are trying to take over the practice of medicine, by setting fees, by deciding what procedures are "medically necessary," by limiting the number of treatment visits, by eliminating coverage for certain conditions, and other measures. In late 2000 the insurance industry in Colorado came within 2 votes of getting legislation passed that would have allowed them to set doctors fees, and would have eliminated "catastrophic claims" which they reported were only 5% of their claims. For most people, the main reason for having insurance is for protection from catastrophes.

In automobile accidents, more and more people are having to hire attorneys to get the medical coverage they have been paying premiums for.

Osteopaths have a special problem with insurance companies. Most insurance companies use the Common Procedural Terminology (C.P.T.) codes established by H.C.F.A. There is one set of codes called Evaluation and Management, with sub-headings of Office Visits for both New Patients, and Established Patients. Then there is a second set of very extensive treatment codes for every medical condition and osteopathic conditions. In medical conditions, once a diagnosis is established, no new evaluation is allowed unless a new medical condition arises. In osteopathic conditions, understanding the structure-function relationship of the body, it is essential to do a structural exam on each visit. Most insurance companies do not understand this at all, not realizing the importance of determining what structural problems exist that are contributing to the patients problems, on established patients what changes have taken place since the last visit, and wouldn't begin to understand that after treatment we do an evaluation to see what we have accomplished with our treatment. This lack of understanding is a particular problem with Medicare.

So what does the future hold? Osteopaths will continue to be world leaders in providing manipulative care for human ills. More and more patients will seek alternatives to traditional medicine. More and more M.D.'s will embrace integrative medicine, but will not understand the real reason the body responds to such methods, and Medicine will change very slowly. Chiropractors will continue to file lawsuits. Insurance companies will continue their efforts to intrude on Medicine.

Section III

Structured (Managed) Health Care

Section III - Table of Contents

16

The Rigid Structure

I n Section II we discussed the structure-function relationship of the human body and how they are inextricably related to each other. Let me stress again that the more rigid the structure, the less functional it becomes, and impaired function inevitably leads to disease. This principle applies just as well to managed or structured health care. The more rigid the structure the less functional it becomes, and therefore leads to significant ills in the health care system. Managed Care was conceived in the 1960's, with the intent of improving the quality of health care, and giving doctors more control over it, with the accent on prevention and maintenance of health. Exactly the opposite has happened. Our health care is poorer, doctors have less control, and too much of available funds is spent on chronic disease.

There are three major problems with Structured Health Care.

First, the myriad of rules and regulations makes a very rigid structure which cannot operate efficiently.

Second , the system suffers from extreme bureaucratic obesity, with so many agencies and organizations involved, all with certain initials, that it has produced an "alphabet soup" (see figure 1, pg. 186) which unlike chicken soup, cures no ills at all.

Third, the major problem is that Structured Health Care functions just like traditional medicine and addresses symptoms, rather than looking for causes.

The superstructure of Managed care, with the endless rules and regulations, requires large numbers of administrators and ancillary workers to operate the system. This requires large sums for salaries, which leaves less for health care itself, and in our present for-profit system, means services must be curtailed or eliminated altogether. These same rules and regulations are damaging the doctor-patient relationship, which is so important in the patient outcome. Doctors are spending increasing amounts of time doing paper work and hassling with redtape, and therefore have less time to spend with patients. All too often they have to restrict services to meet guidelines. Many times they are not allowed to prescribe medications they have found effective, but must use drugs approved by their HMO, or they must substitute generic drugs which are less expensive. In some instances the generic form is as effective as the original, but sometimes they are not. It is my opinion, and that of many others, that most drugs are over-priced. The pharmaceutical industry is a gigantic, powerful, multi-billion dollar industry. Although it is expensive to do the testing to get a drug approved by the Food and Drug Administration (FDA), pharmaceutical companies spend hundreds of millions of dollars each year entertaining doctors and encouraging them to prescribe the company's drugs. They pay "detail persons" to visit doctors offices, inform them about their products, and give them free samples for their own use or to give out to patients. Not too many years ago these representatives were always men, but nowadays they are much more apt to be attractive women. It is an attention-getter.

There are dozens of Medical magazines which are sent to doctors free of charge, which are supported by the drug advertising inside. They contain articles on medical subjects, new technics, and case studies, but are full of page after page of advertising. These magazines must cost additional millions of dollars to print.

As an Osteopathic specialist, many of these magazines are of no particular value in my practice, and concerned about the expense of them and all the trees that have to be cut down to produce the paper, I would write to the publisher and ask to have my name removed from his mailing list. This never worked, but in more recent years I have found a sure-fire way. I take the mailing address with my name and address, mark it "deceased," and mail it to the publisher. That always works.

Managed Care was designed to control the rapidly rising cost of health care and the cost of insurance premiums, by limiting the choice of physicians and by limiting the care or treatment available to only those "medically necessary." Emphasis was to be placed on wellness and prevention, recognizing that chronic conditions cause problems and additional expense. Managed Care was supposed to address three important aspects of health care: cost, access, and quality. The superstructure increases the cost, and in order to make over-all services more widely accessible, some services must be reduced within the framework, and both of these affect the quality. Health care reform also creates more competition, which some do not survive. In the early 1900's there were about a hundred auto manufacturers. Competition has reduced that to three, and Chrysler nearly went under until Lee Iacocca saved the day. Years ago there were neighborhood family run grocery stores, clothing stores, hardware stores, and drug stores. Now competition has wiped them out and they have been replaced by national chains. In all areas of business take-overs and mergers with larger and larger conglomerates, till one can hardly keep up with the changes. The same thing is happening in health care. Small hospitals have gone under. Larger hospitals have been bought by national for-profit management companies. The family doctor, so long revered by so many for his "bedside manner" has been replaced by the Emergency Room and panels of doctors enrolled in HMO's and PPO's.

How do doctors feel about this? In a survey conducted by

Medical Economics *(95)*, doctors ranked managed care as their greatest challenge, and feel it will get worse. Second they ranked loss of autonomy, a by-product of managed care, and feel that it also will get worse. Then they ranked Government intervention, and feel it will get much worse, followed by concern over satisfactory income, again to get much worse. They also voiced concern over incursions by non-physician practitioners, which is another cost-cutting by-product of managed care, and often will lower the level of care. In another survey published in The Denver Post *(96)*, doctors feel that managed care has failed to fulfill the promise of improving preventative care for healthy people. Doctors overwhelmingly view managed care as reducing the quality of care given patients. A survey of 1,100 doctors by the Kaiser Family Foundation found that 9 out of 10 had patients denied coverage for health problems resulting in a serious decline in that patients health, either from denial of medication, or referral to a specialist. This survey covered 400 health care plans, with 70 million patients involved. They stated, "managed care embodies the best and worst in American Medicine. Health plans make decisions based on profit, not patient needs."

Doctors are seeing more conflict between family practitioners and specialists, much due to regulations imposed by HMO's and other management organizations. They feel that what used to be the practice of medicine is now a business venture, with patient care suffering. Doctors strongly feel that they have lost control of medical care, and that the control has been taken over by Managed Care organizations and insurance companies. The feeling is that insurance companies no longer are primarily concerned about the welfare of their clients, but are engaged in the practice of medicine by limiting procedures, by limiting hospital stays, by specifying how many treatments are approved, by denying claims as being "not medically necessary," by reducing payments because of being "over customary charges," and many other intrusions. Because of the many problems, more and more doctors are forced to join larger and larger groups and combines which have more bargaining power. They also join more HMO's and PPO's to get more options. It is not unusual for doctors to belong to 20 or 30 HMO's, and when they sign on they must pay a fee, unlike today's over-paid athletes who receive a multi-million dollar signing bonus when they sign with a team. In addition, most athletes go to college on scholarships, while doctors, both M.D. (Allopathic) and D.O. (Osteopathic) must pay for four years of college, and four years of graduate school. Most then go into a two to five year resident training program during which they are paid, but to finance their earlier education, most have to rely on student loans which must be repaid in funds, or in service in the Armed forces or Public Health. It is not unusual for a doctor to have over $100,000 in a student loan. Still many insurance companies and many people feel that doctors are over-paid. It is interesting to note that Osteopathic doctors consistently have the best record of repaying their student loans.

Many doctors in recent times are turning to Unions to give them more bargaining power. According to a Time article *(97)*, the number of unionized doctors has grown 80% in the last three years. Under present anti-trust laws, only employed doctors can unionize, which is only one out of seven. Some employers maintain that doctors are "supervisors" and therefore not eligible to join unions. In 1999 about 20,000 M.D.'s and D.O.'s were unionized, but legislation to change the anti-trust laws may change that picture significantly. Many doctors, frustrated by all these problems are just retiring from practice long before hey had originally planned. This may help solve the purported over-supply of doctors, but is a poor way to do it.

The massive infra-structure of Managed Care, the accompanying inefficiency, and the decreased revenues of health care providers has created an atmosphere that fosters fraud at all levels. An article in Medical Economics *(98)* "Health Fraud: just business as usual?" cited a New Jersey study which found chiropractors, then Physical Therapists, then Doctors had the highest incidence of fraud. An Insurance fraud task force in Idaho found the same ratio. The General Accounting Office found that California Medicare HMO's were over-paid one billion dollars in 1995. Fraud reaches to the highest levels of Managed Care. An article in the Denver Post *(99)* on July 3, 1999 told about the indictment of several executives of Columbia/HCA Healthcare Corporation, the country's largest hospital chain, having defrauded Medicare and other Government programs out of $3 million. Medicare seems to be a favorite target of fraudulent activities, by organizations, healthcare providers and laboratories. There are a number of instances where fake labs have bilked Medicare of millions. The numbers for healthcare providers are not as large, but nevertheless present. But then when a physician makes an honest mistake, all too often he is accused of fraud. In 1999, Health and Human Services spent $7 million to recruit retired professionals to spot waste, fraud and abuse.

Nurses have big stake in health care. The level of care in hospitals is mainly what is delivered by the nursing staff, some as ordered by staff doctors either M.D. or D.O., but mostly the personal attention they give the patients, the latter a very important ingredient of patient response. With the change from non-profit to for-profit hospitals, the morale of the nursing staff immediately declines because they know the care they give will have to be compromised by cost-cutting measures. Another part of it will be replacing highly trained Registered Nurses by less trained, less paid nurses and aids, which further impairs the level of care. In an article in Physicians Financial News *(100)*, an editorial by Neuro-surgeon Robert White states, "There is a creeping epidemic of a disease of reducing the number of highly trained nurses. It is significantly reducing the quality of health care in this country."

There is also a rapidly growing discontent among patients,

the recipients of health care. Patients feel they are more and more being denied the choice of physicians, choice of procedures, referrals to specialists, and adequate hospital care. At the present time, doctors have an 83% approval rating, which is expected to decline, but patients greatest discontent is with managed care. Formerly their chief worry was "who pays?," but now they worry about getting care at all. Complaints about HMO's have increased 50% in the last three years according to an article in The Rocky Mountain News in 1998 *(101)*. An earlier article in Health Care Observer *(102)* stated that health care recipients see the health care system as disorganized and fraught with greed, waste, and corruption. Based on personal experience, 76% found growing cost the most serious problem, that quality was going downhill, and would continue to do so because of the blind pursuit of profits by insurers and providers. People identified nurses as the key indicator of the quality of care in hospitals, but highly trained nurses were being systematically replaced by poorly trained aids.

Our senior citizens suffer the most from deficiencies in health care, either inherent in the system, or imposed by the restrictions arising from the system. At the present time, seniors comprise about 13% of our population but they use 30% of the prescriptions written, and make up the largest part of health care costs, or more specifically, disease care costs since most of those problems are chronic diseases. Our present health care bill is over a trillion dollars a year. It is estimated that by the year 2020, seniors will comprise 20% of the total population, with that much more added to our oppressive health care bill. At the present time 80% of seniors suffer from one or more degenerative diseases. These are diseases that could be prevented by following the measures outlined in Section I of this book.

Seniors are supposed to be served by Medicare, but many are not. Some cannot afford the premiums, others are deprived of choice of physician. This is particularly true of the Osteopathic profession because of the different philosophies of Allopathic

Medicine, which focuses on symptoms, one organ, or one body part, as opposed to the Osteopathic philosophy which views the whole patient as an integrated unit, which was explained in Section II. Health Care Finance Administration (HCFA), under which Medicare functions, after many conferences with the Osteopathic profession, acknowledges the whole body concept, but then with their Allopathic perspective, divides the body into ten parts - head region, cervical region (neck), thoracic region, lumbar region, sacral region (tail bone), pelvic region (hip bones), lower extremities, upper extremities, rib cage region, abdomen and viscera region (stomach, liver, bowels, etc.). This is a confusing breakdown because the ribs are an integral part of the thoracic area, and by medical dictionary definition, the pelvis includes the hip bones and the sacrum. So much for bureaucratic intelligence. HCFA allows certain remuneration for each body part. As a part of Medicare, doctors are also allowed remuneration for "Evaluation and Management" (E & M), and then is sub-divided into office visits for new, or established patients. For medical cases, once a diagnosis has been arrived at, for instance hypertension, then no further E & M charges are allowed unless some new condition arises and further evaluation is necessary. In Osteopathic practice it is much different though. Even though it is not always necessary to treat all ten body areas, with more complicated cases it often is. In any case it is always important to examine the whole body on each visit to determine if there are any dysfunctions present which may be contributing to the patients problems, and if found what the best method of manipulative treatment is indicated. In some states, Medicare simply cannot comprehend this, Colorado where I live being one of the worst. I will with-hold judgement, but several years ago, a former Director of Payor Relations of the American Osteopathic Association, whose job it was to handle Medicare and other third party payor problems, accused the Colorado Director of Medicare of being prejudiced. I will quote a letter by a patient of mine who was denied coverage under Medicare, and took the time to write and complain. "Dear Mrs. "Doe," "Your letter has been referred to me for response. After reviewing your letter regarding your Osteopathic Doctor we took these issues to our Medical Director." This is the summarization of his response. "First, Medicare is regulated by Health Care Finance Administration. We have had extensive communication with the central office of Medicare with the national office of the American Osteopathic Association on this matter. The local Osteopath is wrong in his interpretation of the regulation." (Note: I used the guidelines published by the American Osteopathic Association).

"Second, Medicare understands the 'whole body' concept of osteopathic manipulation. However, Medicare believes that whole body manipulation is not always 'medically necessary' to treat the patient's condition. On many occasions a limited treatment to one or two areas is sufficient." (Note: the problem in this instance was not the number of areas, but the denial of E & M charges, and the reason for treating multiple areas was fully documented).

"This carrier regrets any inconvenience it may have caused this physician, but it believes that the physicians practice was significantly at variance with Medicare policy and needs to be adjusted." (Note: again, I used guidelines published by the American Osteopathic Association after numerous conferences with HCFA).

One of the problems that all doctors have with Medicare is that claims are paid, and then reviewed in retrospect. Occasionally this uncovers fraud, in many instances proves to be adequate, but if the physician has made an error, or the auditing clerk has made an error or mis-interprets the guidelines, the doctor is forced to refund money or face stiff fines and jail sentences. According to an article in Government and Medicine *(103)* mistakes by auditors are quite frequent. Appeals are quite costly, not only in the legal fees involved, but in the time taken out of the office, which many doctors, believe it or not , do not feel they can afford.

Another problem with Medicare is it's direct contradiction of it's expressed purpose - to lower the cost of health care. Until 1998, patients under Medicare coverage could not pay out of pocket for health care services. National surveys showed that about 15% of patients could afford to pay for such services, which would have saved the Government a significant sum. Now doctors can let patients pay out of pocket, but they must sign an agreement not to see other Medicare patients for two years. That makes no sense at all.

The second major problem which I have termed "bureaucratic obesity" is that managed care has spawned an unbelievable number of agencies and designations with long names which must be abbreviated as letters, creating the "alphabet soup." This again increases the cost of health care requiring cuts in services provided, more paper work, and more frustration for doctors. This "alphabet soup" is outlined in *figure 1* (following page). I am sure the list is far from complete.

The major problem with Managed or Structured Health Care is that in addressing the cost, the same approach is used as in traditional medicine, symptoms are addressed and not the causes. The United States has by far the most costly health care system, but not the best. This is not to say that we have not made some extraordinary technological advances, but our over-all health care ranks below many other countries. A study by the Organization for Economic Cooperation and Development *(104)* showed the average cost of health care in the U.S. was $3,094 per person which was 13.6 % of our Gross Domestic Product. Of 23 other countries, all were 8.1% or less. They found the U.S. 5th in infant mortality, and highest in low birth weight babies. A study in the 1980's by the World Health Organization, which included all of the organized countries in the world, studied mortality statistics, morbidity, time loss from work, time loss from school, etc. The U.S. had the 4th highest per capita income, the eighth high-

AAHP	American Association of Health Plans.
AFL-CIO	American Federation of Labor - Congress of Industrial Organizations.
AFSCME	American Federation of State, County & Municipal Employees.
AMGA	American Medical Group Association.
DRG's	Diagnosis Related Groups.
ERISA	Employees Retirement Income Security Act.
HCFA	Health Care Finance Administration.
HHS	Health and Human Services.
HMO	Health Maintenance Organization.
ICD-9-CM	International Classification of Disease, 9th revision, Clinical Modification.
IPA	Independent Physicians Association.
LPN	Licensed Practical Nurse.
MCO	Managed Care Organizations.
NAMM	North American Medical Management.
NA	Nurses Aide.
NP	Nurse Practitioner.
OPEIU	Office of Professional Employees International Union.
PCP	Primary Care Physician.
PHO	Physician-Hospital Organization.
PMC	Physician Management Company.
POD	Physician Organization Delivery (system).
PPM	Physician Practice Management (companies).
PPO	Preferred Provider Organization.
PSN	Provider Service Network.
PSO	Provider Sponsored Organization
SEIU	Service Employees International Union.

(Figure 1)

est number of doctors, the most food (such as it was) available, but ranked 42nd in level of health. This is a very poor testimonial. During the Second World War 50% of draft age men were found unfit for military duty, ones that were supposed to be in the prime of life.

All of the "solutions" being presented so far to solve the cost of health care, involve more regulations, more bureaucracy, and more Governmental regulation. This has proven to be anything but successful. The answer lies in two major changes in the practice of medicine. Emphasis must truly be placed on prevention, not "preventative" drugs, but on preventative health habits which "The Father of Medicine," Hippocrates advocated, and as has been outlined in Section I of this book. The second, a monumental task, but absolutely necessary to achieve the desired goal, is to change the way doctors are taught and how they practice. They must get away from the Cnidian Philosophy of focusing on symptoms, and embrace the Hippocratic Holistic Philosophy. The most important part of that is the time-honored art of physical diagnosis, which most doctors have lost, or in recent years have not been taught. Dr. Robert H. Ebert, former Dean of Harvard Medical School, pointed out over a decade ago that "Health Centers, operating rooms, and modern diagnostic technics are a part of but not the essence of Medicine." *(105)* Doctors have been seduced by our high tech advances in diagnostic equipment, such as Magnetic Resonance Imaging, Ultrasound, Computed Tomography, Nuclear Medicine, and sophisticated lab procedures. An MRI is around $1000, and $50 to $100 more with contrast media. A CT Scan of the brain runs between $250 to $800. The Mayo Brothers became famous because they were so good at physical diagnosis, and built their reputation on the ability to accurately diagnose problems and then appropriately treat them. Even that venerable institution has succumbed to the lure of our dramatic, high tech, expensive diagnostic devices. These devices have been very helpful, and can be very revealing, but there are many instances when a careful physical examination would make an expensive MRI not necessary. I had one patient with chronic low back pain who had been subjected to nine MRI's at $1000 a session. She was a teacher, and was on her feet all day long. Physical diagnosis revealed a short right leg which kept her pelvis out of balance resulting in a chronic inflammation of the sciatic nerve. A heel lift and manipulative treatment corrected the problem. A number of years ago the Radiation Division of the Food and Drug Administration concluded that 40% of X-rays were unnecessary, and probably in reality the figure was higher than that. The same figures undoubtedly apply to our more sophisticated procedures.

Laboratory tests have also become more sophisticated and expensive, but again a careful physical diagnosis would often eliminate the need for such tests, or narrow them down to one or two to confirm a diagnosis. Several years ago I was riding on a ski tow with a young lady lab technician from Milwaukee. In the course of our conversation she said her pet peeve was doing lab work and having the doctor standing in the door waiting for her to make a diagnosis.

Physical diagnosis involves four basic procedures, viz. inspection, percussion, auscultation, and palpation.

Inspection. A great deal can be learned about a patient by simply observing them. Their general appearance, facial expression, posture, gait, body symmetry, skin, the look in their eyes. This can give the doctor much valuable information about the patient.

Percussion. "Thumping" various parts of the body can give helpful information about body contents, and differences between gases, liquids, and solid tissues. This can often eliminate or reduce the need for diagnostic tests.

Auscultation. This basic skill is still practiced by most doctors, and can give important information about the heart, lungs, bowels, and blood vessels. It can be enhanced by our modern technology, but should not be replaced by it.

Palpation. This is the most important and most neglected aspect of physical diagnosis, and where the greatest void exits. Palpation has been a part of patient examination as long as recorded medical history, which goes back to ancient Egypt. In Egyptian medical hierarchy, there were the priest-physician, the surgeon and veterinary, the ever-present magician, and the bandagists, who wrapped the mummies. Only the priest-physician was allowed to touch the patient, stated thusly: "I am chief of the priests, chief of the magicians, chief physician to the king, who everyday reads the books, who treats the sick, who lays his hand on the diseased, whereby he knows them; gifted in the examination with the hand." *(105)*

Careful palpation of the patient reveals a great deal about all aspects of the patient. Osteopathic Physicians receive extensive training in palpation and many achieve high degrees of skill in this area, but as outlined in Section II, some have neglected their training and just practice traditional medicine. Palpation reveals the state of health or severity of disease, the presence of fever, evidence of trauma and even the direction the trauma was inflicted in the body, the presence of undue stress, whether or not the patient is eating properly especially in protein intake, whether or not the patient is getting adequate exercise, evidence of postural habits, the presence of occupational strains, and the patients energy level. The texture of the soft tissues is changed in alcoholism, in diabetes, and in infections. The manner in which palpation is done is important in the doctor-patient relationship. It is important to be gentle, and patients can tell whether or not the doctor is competent, knowledgeable and thorough. As discussed in Section II, Osteopathic physical diagnosis also involves investigation of many reflex phenomena which gives very valuable information about not only the neuro-musculo-skeletal system, but the state of the internal organs. In many instances this reveals information about the body that not even the most sophisticated imaging procedures can show. This can make a significant saving in the cost of health care.

For many years the medical community derided Osteopathic palpation and manipulative treatment as the "laying on of hands," but now with the clinical success of Osteopathy, the extensive research which has proven the philosophy, and with other approaches such as Delores Krieger's Therapeutic Touch, the therapeutic value of a hands-on approach is more widely accepted, but not utilized as it should be.

My father had this to say about palpation in his book, "Osteopathy in the Cranial Field," *(77)* which as Osteopathy spreads throughout the world, has been translated into French, German, Italian, and Japanese. "The human hand has been called the greatest single diagnostic instrument known to man. Marvelous as the advances of objective science may be, nothing takes the place of a searching analysis of the tissues with a well-trained palpatory sense, to determine not only the condition present but the best procedure to modify it. This is a study from the aspect of function, not stasis; living physiology, not cadaveric anatomy. The X-ray may show gross changes in pathology; the laboratory, alterations in chemistry; but neither can reveal the fine shades of tissue tone and tension, mobility, elasticity, resiliency, flexibility, extensibility, reaction to stimuli and all the other things so essential to adequate diagnosis." The art of physical diagnosis, with special emphasis on palpation of tissues must be re-instated in our Medical Schools. This will significantly reduce the necessity of many expensive diagnostic procedures, and add considerable information about the patient's condition.

Another important change must take place, and that is universal understanding and acceptance of "alternative medicine." This is defined as "anything not taught in American Medical Schools." This includes a vast, confusing list of alternative choices, many time-honored, others just now proving themselves. This would include Osteopathic manipulation as explained in Section II, acupuncture and Chinese Medicine which have been in use for about 5,000 years, Ayurvedic Medicine, Chiropractic, Herbal Medicine, Homeopathy, Naturopathy, Reflexology, Shiatsu, and numerous types of manual therapy. In the last several decades there has been a significant increased awareness of the importance of the neuro-musculo-skeletal system as a source of pain and disability. This has produced a great array of hands-on therapies, and much wider utilization of them in approaching health problems. The exclusion of these many therapies from Medical practice is changing. Almost one third of our Medical Schools now offer courses in Alternative Therapies, and the American Medical Association is encouraging it's members to become better informed on the subject. In 1995 the American Medical Association established a task force to explore the inclusion of "manual medicine" in the curriculum of Medical Schools. There is an excellent book on Alternative Medicine, and how to choose an appropriate therapy by Mary and Michael Morton. *(106)* In 1998 in Denver, Kenton Johnson published a booklet, titled "Complementary Healing," listing practitioners of alternative healing who desired to be listed in the booklet. He has now expanded it to a web site. (107)

17

Solutions

F or many years the constant criticism from the Medical
Profession about Osteopathy was "there is no scientific
proof," even though Osteopathy was very successful clinically.
Eventually the research was accomplished which substantiated the Osteopathic Philosophy, not only in this country, but
by scientists in other countries as well. We have heard the
same criticism about many alternative methods, but in recent
years much of that smoke screen has been dissipated by extensive, valid research of many kinds. I have wondered for
many years if traditional medicine could stand the test of "scientific proof." There is a story about a dowager who went to
her meat market to get a stewing chicken for a special dinner
she was giving. She asked the butcher to let her examine the
chicken. She poked it, squeezed it, sniffed it and said it
wouldn't do. The butcher produced a second chicken which
received the same examination, and was also rejected. The
butcher produced a third chicken which the lady poked,
squeezed, and sniffed under each wing, and again rejected.
The butcher then said, "lady, could you pass that test?"

Could traditional medicine pass tests of scientific proof?
At the present time, well over 160,000 persons a year die from

prescription medicines. This is accepted as part of the practice of medicine. About 20% of hospital admissions are due to drug reactions. Of drug-related emergency room visits, 60% are for prescription drugs. Mistakes on prescriptions, either by the doctor or by the pharmacist account for 30,000 deaths a year. Millions of unnecessary surgeries are performed each year, with an estimated 50,000 fatalities. The implementation of "second opinion" has not reduced these figures significantly. The incidence of hospital induced infections has reached serious proportions because hospitals must cut corners, reduce services, they become lax in enforcing sterile procedures, and in some instances they suppress reports on the problem.

There are over 500,000 by-pass surgeries done each year, which some medical experts claim are unnecessary. The average cost of such surgery is $40,000, and in 5 years 50% of those patients have clogged arteries again, and in 7 years 80% do. Many of these heart problems could be avoided or cured by proper nutrition.

The incidence of otitis media (inner ear infection) has increased over 200% in the last 20 years. The medical profession itself attributes much of this to over-prescribing antibiotics. Also a part of the problem is more working mothers with children in day-care where they are constantly exposed to infections from other children.

In spite of great technical advances, our American health care system (the most expensive in the world) has many deficiencies, and in the light of how they judge others, does not fare very well. Many of those deficiencies could be corrected.

What can we do in this regard? First and foremost, take charge of your health. Be the master of your fate and the captain of your soul. Change your life-style as outlined in Section I. It takes will-power, but it can be done. Too few people appreciate their health until they start losing it. Secondly, avail yourself of alternative methods, which often have much to offer. All too often you are told to take a pill of one kind or another for every ailment that comes along. Make no mistake though, there is a big difference between vitamin pills and medicine pills. When a medicine is prescribed for you, always with possible side-effects, ask yourself, "is there a more natural, safe way to address this problem?" Most of the time there is.

Thirdly, voice your dissatisfaction when you are denied your choice of a doctor, especially when you want one that uses a holistic approach. Voice your dissatisfaction when you are denied treatment that has proven to be helpful, especially when you are told "there is no scientific proof," or it is "not medically necessary." Insurance companies are more and more taking control of the practice of Medicine and Osteopathy in order to increase their profits. Have you heard of any insurance company going bankrupt? I haven't.

More and more we are being told, "We will think for you," "Big Brother is looking out for you," "Big Government will take care of you," You can do a better job yourself, knowing what to do. Take charge of your life like Norman Cousins did *(53)*. Demand your own holistic doctor, demand better hospital care.

We hear a great deal about "preventative medicine." Many drugs are prescribed to prevent certain diseases, but all too often they cause other diseases. The index of Iatrogenic Diseases (doctor caused diseases) is getting bigger each year. Aspirin is considered a safe drug and is prescribed for the prevention of heart attacks, but 5,000 people a year die from taking aspirin, usually those taking large doses, Hearts can be kept healthy with good nutrition. The best prevention of all is keeping your body healthy through nutrition, exercise, sleep, etc., and keeping it normal structurally, which will allow it to function normally. Exercise will help improve the structure-function relationship of the body, but the best thing is regular Osteopathic treatment.

Lastly, make your feelings known to your elected officials. Some of them listen, and if enough people bring enough pressure to bear, some changes can be accomplished. So in all these areas, be the "Master of your fate and the Captain of your soul."

Good health to you.

BIBLIOGRAPHY

(ibid) Refers to the previous reference number.

(1) Encyclopedia Britannica, Inc., Micropedia, 15th Edition, Pg. 1020.

(2) "Let's Get Well." Adelle Davis.
Harcourt, Brace and World, Inc. Pg. 148.

(3) "Eat Right for Your Type." Dr. Peter D'Adamo.
G.P. Putnam's Sons.

(4) American Journal of Public Health. 1996: 86 (12) 1729.

(5) "Losing It: America's Obsession With Weight and the Industry That Feeds On It." Laura Fraser. Dutton.

(6) The Environmental Working Group. Dr. John Folts.
University of Wisconsin School of Medicine.

(7) "Spontaneous Healing." Andrew Weil, M.D.
Alfred A. Knopf, Inc.

(8) "Nutrition Breakthrough." Robert Atkins, M.D.
William Morrow & Co.

(9) "Health Revelations." Robert Atkins, M.D.
Agora Health Publishing. Baltimore.

(10) "Second Opinion." William C. Douglas, M.D.
Second Opinion Publishing. Atlanta.

(11) "Health and Healing." Julian Whitaker, M.D.
Whitaker's Wellness Institute. Newport Beach.

(12) "Arthritis and Common Sense." Dale Alexander.
Simon and Scheuster.

(13) "Do You really Need Glasses?" Marilyn Rosanes-Berrett, Ph.D. Published by Author.

(14) "Macbeth." William Shakespeare. Scene II.

(15) Textbook of Medical Physiology. Guyton and Hall. W. B. Saunders Co.

(16) "The Coming Plague." Laurie Garrett. Farrar, Straus and Giroux. New York.

(17) "Imprimins." Hillsdale College. Vol. 27 #10. Oct. 1998.

(18) "Clinical Pearl News." I.T. Services. Vol. 9, No. 7. July 1999.

(19) USA Weekend. Jan. 3-5, 1997.

(20) Frank Willard, Ph.D. New England College of Osteopathic Medicine. Lecture AAO, 1997.

(21) "The Power of Positive Thinking." Norman Vincent Peale. Foundation for Christian Living.

(22) Medical and Health Annual 1996. Encyclopedia Britannica, Inc. Pg. 369.

(23) Medical and Health Annual 1997. Encyclopedia Britannica Inc. Pg. 287.

(24) "Depression." Parade Magazine. September 26, 1997.

(25) "A Physical Finding Related to Psychiatric Disorders." John Woods, D.O. & Rachel Woods, D.O. Journal of American Osteopathic Association. August 1961.

(26) "Treating the Body, Healing the Mind." Hippocrates Magazine. April 1997.

(27) "Love, Medicine and Miracles." Bernie S. Seigal, M.D. Harper and Row.

(28) "Can Prayer Heal?" Hippocrates Magazine. April 1998.

(29) "Faith and Healing." Time Magazine. June 24, 1996.

(30) "If Longevity is Your Goal, Go To Church." Rocky Mountain News. May 19, 1999.

(31) Viola Frymann, D.O., F.A.A.O. Personal correspondence.

(32) I. M. Korr, Ph.D. Director of Research and Professor Emeritus of Physiology. Kirksville College of Osteopathic Medicine.

(33) Robert Wood Johnson Foundation. Researched by Brandies University. Rocky Mountain News. October 22, 1993.

(34) "The Paradox of Smoking." Richard L. Crowther, FAIA. A.B. Hirshfield Press. 1983.

(35) "Passive Smoke Doubles Heart Risk." The Denver Post. May 20, 1997.

(36) "Parent Smoking Kills 6,200 Kids." The Denver Post. July 15, 1997.

(37) "Smoking Costs." Bottom Line. June 15, 1990. Vol. 11 #11. Boardroom, Inc.

(38) "Osteopathic Medicine Holds Solution in Healthcare Crisis." Harold Magoun Jr. D.O., F.A.A.O. The D.O May 1995. The American Osteopathic Association.

(39) "Kicking the Habit." The D.O. April 1996. The American Osteopathic Association.

(40) "College Crisis: Booze Before Books." Carnegie Foundation. Encyclopedia Britannica Yearbook, 1998.

(41) "DUI Arrests Up for Third Year." The Denver Post. July 28, 1999.

(42) "The French Paradox." Modern Medicine. Vol. 63. April 1995.

(43) "Second Opinion." William Campbell Douglas, M.D. Vol. IX No. 7. July 1999.

(44) "The Natural Mind." Andrew Weil, M.D. Houghton Mifflin Co. Boston.

(45) "Silent Spring." Rachel Carson. Houghton Mifflin Co. Boston.

(46) "Indoor Air: Risks and Remedies." Richard L. Crowther, FAIA. Published by Author.

(47) "Genetically Altered Food." U.S. News and World Reports. July 26, 1999.

(48) "High Tech Farming." The Denver Post. July 31, 1999.

(49) "The Greatest Benefit to Mankind." Roy Porter. W. W. Norton & Co. 1997.

(50) "The Story of Medicine." Victor Robinson. The New Home Library. 1931.

(51) "Divided Legacy: The Conflict Between the Homeopathy and the AMA." Harris Coulter. North Atlantic Books. 1982.

(52) Encyclopedia Britannica. 15th Edition. William Benton. 1943-73.

(53) "Anatomy of an Illness as Perceived by the Patient." Norman Cousins. W. W. Norton & Co. 1979.

(54) "Love, Medicine, and Miracles." Bernie Siegal, M.D. Harper & Row. 1986.

(55) "Timeless Healing." Herbert Benson, M.D. Scribner Publishing Co. 1996

(56) "Spontaneous Healing." Andrew Weil, M.D. Alfred Knopf, N.Y. 1995

(57) "Autobiography of Andrew Taylor Still." Published by Author. 1908

(58) "The Household Physician." Ira Warren, A.M., M.D. Bradley Dayton Co. Boston 1862

(59) "Frontier Doctor, Medical Pioneer." Charles E. Still Jr., D.O. Thomas Jefferson University Press at Northeast Missouri State University. Kirksville, MO. 1991

(60) "History of Osteopathy." E. R. Booth, Ph. D., D.O. Press of Jennings and Graham. Cincinnati. 1905

(61) "The First School of Osteopathic Medicine." Georgia Warner Walter. Thomas Jefferson University Press at Northeast Missouri State University. Kirksville, MO 1992

(62) "Philosophy of Osteopathy." Andrew Taylor Still. Kirksville, MO 1899.

(63) "The Lengthening Shadow of Dr. Andrew Taylor Still." Arthur G. Hildreth, D.O. Published by Author. Macon, MO 1938.

(64) "Take It From a D.C. - a lot of Chiropractic is a Sham." Medical Economics. September 17, 1990.

(65) "My Most Unforgettable Character." Harold Magoun, Sr. D.O., F.A.A.O. The D.O. April, 1973.

(66) "Studies in the Osteopathic Sciences." Louisa Burns, M.S., D.O., D.S.O. The Occident Printing, Los Angeles 1907. Vol. 1. Basic Principles. Vol. 2. The Nerve Centers. Vol. 3. The Physiology of Consciousness. Vol. 4. Cells of the Blood.

(67) "The Reflex Activity in the Spinal Extensors." Denslow and Clough. Journal of Neuro-physiology, 1941.

(68) "Axonal Transport, Trophic Function of Nerves." I. M. Korr, Ph.D. The Collected Papers of I. M. Korr. American Academy of Osteopathy Year Book. 1979.

(69) "Osteopathic Perspectives: Medical History." Michael Kuchera, D.O., F.A.A.O. Kirksville College of Osteopathic Medicine. 1995.

(70) "Osteopathic Mechanisms." Edythe Ashmore, D.O. Journal Printing Co. Kirksville. 1915.

(71) "Osteopathic Technics." Ernest E. Tucker, D.O. Clinton Press. New York. 1917.

(72) "Osteopathic Strap Technic." Joseph Swart. D.O., LL.B. Kansas City. 1923.

(73) "Splenic Stimulation." Yale Castlio and Louise Ferris-Smith. AAO Yearbook. 1955.

(74) "Symptoms of Visceral Disease." Francis Pottenger, M.D., FACP, C.V. Mosby Co. St. Louis, MO. 1919.

(75) "With Thinking Fingers." Adah Strand Sutherland. The Cranial Academy. 1962.

(76) "Familiar Quotations." John Bartlett. Little Brown and Co. Boston, Toronto, London. 1992.

(77) "Osteopathy in the Cranial Field." Harold Magoun, Sr., D.O., F.A.A.O. Journal Printing Co. Kirksville, MO. 1951, 1966, 1976.

(78) "Self Healing." Andrew Weil, M.D. Thorne Communications, Inc. 42 Pleasant St., Watertown, MA.

(79) "Sinus Survival." Dr. Robert S. Ivker, Jeremy P. Tarcher, Inc. Los Angeles. 1991.

(80) "Osteopathic Manipulation in a Hospital Environment." Edward Stiles, D.O., F.A.A.O. American Academy of Osteopathy Yearbook. 1977.

(81) "A Physical Finding Related to Psychiatric Disorders." John M. Woods, D.O., Rachel H. Woods, D.O., JAOA. August 1961.

(82) "Relationship of Disturbances of the Cranio-Sacral Mechanism to Symptomatology of the Newborn," Viola M. Frymann, D.O., F.A.A.O. JAOA. 1966.

(83) "Otitis Media, an Osteopathic Approach." Alistair Moresi, Bach. App. Sc. (Osteopathy), The Cranial Letter, Vol. 50, #3.

(84) "My Basketball Bible." Forrest C. Allen, D.O. Smith-Grieves Co. Kansas City. 1924.

(85) "Myofascial Manipulative Release of Carpal Tunnel Syndrome: Documentation with MRI." Benjamin M. Sucher, D.O., JAOA Vol. 93, #12. 1993.

(86) "Webster's Third New International Dictionary." Encyclopedia Britannica. 1971.

(87) "The Denver Post." June 21, 2000. News Day.

(88) "Physicians Desk Reference." Medical Economics Co., Inc. Montvale, NJ.

(89) "Health Revelations." Dr. Robert Atkins. April, 1999.

(90) "The Story of Medicine." Victor Robinson, M.D. The New Home Library. 1931.

(91) "Arthritis Today." Arthritis Foundation. 1330 West Peachtree. Atlanta, GA.

(92) "The D.O." American Osteopathic Association. Vol. 41 #10.

(93) "Self Healing." Andrew Weil, M.D. December, 2000.

(94) "Stedman's Medical Dictionary." 25th Edition. Williams & Wilkins, A Waverly Co.

(95) "You're Hassled, Here's Why." Medical Economics. October 19, 1998.

(96) "Docs See HMO's as Impediment." Denver Post. July 29, 1999.

(97) "Unionizing the E.R." Time Magazine. July 5, 1999.

(98) "Health Fraud: Just Business as Usual." Medical Economics. July 10, 1995.

(99) "Columbia Execs Convicted of Fraud." The Denver Post. July 3, 1999.

(100) "Editorial." Physicians Financial News. Vol. 15 #10. July 19, 1997.

(101) "Complaints Against HMO's." Rocky Mountain News. October 11, 1998.

(102) "Consumers Bash Hospitals, Health Plans." Health Care Observer. Vol. 2 #7. July, 1997.

(103) "Post-payment Audits Rankle Physicians." Government and Medicine. December 14, 1998.

(104) Organization for Economic Cooperation and Development. October 4, 1994.

(105) "Medical Health Annuals." Encyclopedia Britannica. 1997.

(106) "Five Steps to Selecting the Best Alternative Medicine." Mary and Michael Morton. New World Library. 1996.

(107) Kenton Johnson. www.CompWellness.com.

STRUCTURED HEALING

ADDENDUM

This addition to my book became necessary when just after I had sent my book to the printer, I became aware of a stunning advance in nutrition.

As an Osteopathic Physician I was taught that the body is able to heal itself, as taught by Andrew Taylor Still, M.D., founder of Osteopathy in the 1860's and 70's. Then when my mother, expected to die of tubercular glomerulonephritis (kidney disease) was restored to health by Adelle Davis, nutritional program, I became acutely aware of the importance of nutrition in health. Practicing these two vital philosophies for 50 years, I have seen many dramatic responses to my treatment. But I have been frustrated by only providing partial help many difficult cases of severe degenerative disease, chronic fibromyalgia, multiple sclerosis, osteoporosis, cancer, etc. That has changed.

A recent patient of mine, Mr. Ferris Haddad, introduced me to Mannatech, a new company formed in Dallas in 1994. Mr. Haddad has been teaching nutrition to doctors, their patients, athletes, and their trainers for over 20 years. Mannatech instantly appealed to him, and he joined the company. He has recruited some of the top medical specialists and researchers for Mannatech, and is a Platinum Presidential Director of the company.

Mannatech's research, and information based on the research of other scientists, has found that of the 200 carbohydrates identified so far, a well known source of energy, there are 8 special carbohydrates that are absolutely essential for cell communication and function. They are mannose, galactose, fucose (not fructose), xylose, glucose, sialic acid,

N-acetylglucosamine, and N-acetylgalactosamine. These glycoproteins act as receptors on the surface of mammalian cells and also on invading pathogens. Mannose appears to block the receptor sites on pathogens and thus prevent infections. This newly discovered cell communication is absolutely essential for normal cell function. In the past several years, two of the Nobel Prizes in Medicine and Physiology have been for research in cell communication.

To illustrate how important communication is, let me cite an example on a much larger scale. The Gulf War was the shortest and most successful military campaign in history. The primary target of the U. S. Military and it's allies was Iraq's communication system, which was almost entirely destroyed by the initial strikes. Without communication the Iraq military was totally ineffective. Without cell communication, our bodily functions are equally ineffective.

Our modern diets are lacking most of these 8 essential glycoproteins, so it is no wonder that our level of health has declined in the last 2 generations. Most of our foods are grown on depleted soils, are artificially fertilized, are picked green before they can manufacture vital nutrients and so they can be shipped 100's or 1000's of miles with a minimum of spoilage. In addition they are treated with insecticides, and are now being genetically altered.

Mannatech has almost 100 patents involving the extraction, concentration and preservation of these vital nutrients from vine-ripened foods, which then allow the body to function normally as it was designed. This allows the body to overcome almost any disease, many which are now considered "incurable." Mannatech is rapidly spreading world-wide both by word-of-mouth and by a networking system. Information can be obtained on their website:

www.mannatech-inc.com